Hormones and Metabolic Control

A medical student's guide to control of various aspects
of normal and abnormal metabolism

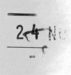

Preface

We feel it essential that medical students have a firm grasp not only of basic biochemical principles but also of sophisticated interactions of hormones in the control of intermediary metabolism. Present medical courses attempt to illustrate such control with a variety of ordered and disordered metabolic states. The stimulus for writing this book came from discussions with many of our own medical students who had difficulty in finding suitable texts covering regulatory aspects of biochemistry. This situation became particularly apparent when one of us (M.B.) embarked on the medical course here in Nottingham.

Use of the present text assumes that the reader has access to standard text books of biochemistry and physiology. No attempt has been made to describe in detail the steps of intermediary metabolism and no structural formulae have been included. Chapter one and the Appendix are introductory and serve to cover the actions of hormones at molecular and metabolic levels, giving brief descriptions of important regulatory sites in intermediary metabolism. This information is used in subsequent chapters to describe and analyse a variety of normal and abnormal metabolic states. In this way we hope that the book will serve as a useful text for students at the second M.B. level and also for junior clinical students, providing a bridge between preclinical and formal clinical teaching.

We are grateful to colleagues at the Queen's Medical Centre, Nottingham for helpful discussion during the writing of the book and to Marie Caunt for typing the original manuscript so clearly and quickly. We also wish to thank Dr Judith Bradshaw for help in proof-reading.
1984

David A. White
Bruce Middleton
Michael Baxter

Hormones and Metabolic Control

A medical student's guide to control of various aspects of normal and abnormal metabolism

David A. White

BSc, PhD
Senior Lecturer, Department of Biochemistry, University of Nottingham
Medical School

Bruce Middleton

MA, PhD
Lecturer, Department of Biochemistry, University of Nottingham Medical
School

Michael Baxter

BSc, BMedSci, PhD
Faculty of medicine,
University of Nottingham Medical School

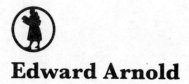

Edward Arnold

© David A. White, Bruce Middleton and Michael Baxter 1984

First published 1984
by Edward Arnold (Publishers) Ltd
41 Bedford Square
London WC1B 3DQ

British Library Cataloguing in Publication Data

White, David A.
  Hormones and metabolic control.
  1. Hormones—Physiological effect
  2. Metabolic regulation
  I. Title   II. Middleton, Bruce
  III. Baxter, Michael
  612'.405   QP571

ISBN 0-7131-4437-8   18/10/84

Whilst the advice and information in this book is believed to be true and accurate at
the date of going to press, neither the authors nor the publisher can accept any legal
responsibility or liability for any errors or omissions that may be made.

Text set in Monophoto Baskerville
Printed and Bound in Great Britain by
Butler & Tanner Ltd, Frome and London

Contents

Normal energy metabolism and its control

This chapter attempts a brief overview of the process of energy metabolism (the breakdown and synthesis of storage forms) and its control in man. Metabolism can be defined as the sum of the chemical changes constantly occurring in a living cell. It can be divided into two fundamental processes: *anabolism*, those changes involving the biosynthesis of cell macromolecules and *catabolism*, the breakdown of complex molecules to provide energy (in the form of ATP and reducing equivalents) for cell function and to provide precursors for anabolism. Thus, because anabolism requires simultaneous catabolism, the process of catabolism has to be directed and controlled to avoid wasteful degradation of newly synthesized material. Also since cells and tissues can exist for limited periods in a catabolic state, the anabolic processes are likewise subject to control. The balance between the anabolic and the catabolic state in man is achieved by the actions of hormones in co-ordinating and controlling tissue responses. The control of these responses can be acute (occurring over a period of minutes or less) or chronic (occurring over hours or days). Chronic control affects amounts of enzymes while acute control involves rapid modification of the activity of existing enzyme molecules. These two modes of control allow the tissue to adapt its metabolism via the chronic effect to changes initially imposed as a result of acute effects (Fig. 1.1).

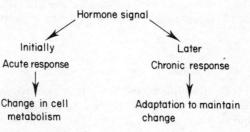

Fig. 1.1   Tissue response to hormone signals.

Catabolism

The hormonal profile typifying this state is one in which the plasma concentration of insulin is lowered while the concentration of adrenaline, glucagon, glucocorticoids and growth hormone is elevated (Table 1.1). Insulin can be regarded as anabolic in overall effect while the other hormones mentioned above are generally catabolic in effect. An important factor in determining the 'set' of metabolism is the ratio of these two groups of hormones, but the magnitude of any specific tissue responses to a hormone depends on its concentration and the relative number of receptors at the site of action.

Table 1.1　Hormonal changes in metabolic states

Anabolism		Catabolism	
Hormonal changes	*Metabolic effects*	*Hormonal changes*	*Metabolic effects*
Insulin　↑	Increased formation of protein, glycogen and triglyceride.	Insulin　↓	Increased mobilization and breakdown of glucose, fatty acids and amino acids liberated from tissue stores (glycogen, triglyceride and protein)
Glucagon　↓		Glucagon　↑	
Adrenaline　↓		Adrenaline　↑	
Cortisol　↓		Cortisol　↑	
(Glucocorticoids)		(Glucocorticoids)	
Growth hormone　↑*	Increased synthesis of fatty acids and sterols	Growth hormone　↑*	

* Elevation of growth hormone in the presence of raised insulin concentrations is anabolic in effect, but is catabolic when insulin levels are decreased and cortisol levels raised.

Fat catabolism

This can be divided into two phases: mobilization of free fatty acids (FFA) from triglyceride (TG) and oxidation of the resulting acyl-groups yielding acetyl-CoA.

Mobilization

The largest store of triglyceride occurs in white adipose tissue but the subsequent metabolism of fatty acids released from stores occurs in liver, heart, kidney and skeletal muscle (Fig. 1.2). This is because white adipose tissue does not have a high capacity for FFA oxidation (unlike brown adipose tissue which can rapidly oxidize fatty acids to produce heat, see Chapter 6). In all types of adipose tissue the enzyme regulating lipolysis is the triglyceride lipase which catalyses the removal of the first acyl-group. This enzyme is activated acutely by phosphorylation which occurs as a consequence of raised cAMP concentrations and activation of a protein kinase. Growth hormone

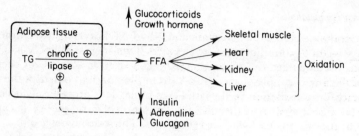

Fig. 1.2 Mobilization of fatty acids.

and glucocorticoid cause a more chronic stimulation of TG lipase by increasing the amount of enzyme.

Fatty acid oxidation

Tissue uptake and subsequent metabolism of FFA is controlled by its concentration in blood. In liver incoming fatty acyl-units partition between oxidation and TG reformation (Fig. 1.3). The distribution depends on the

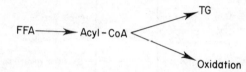

Fig. 1.3 Liver response to plasma FFA.

exact hormonal status. In the majority of catabolic situations β-oxidation predominates but in cases of peripheral insulin resistance (e.g. injury) TG resynthesis in liver can be more important. In other tissues incoming fatty acids are usually β-oxidized. Fatty acid oxidation occurs primarily by β-oxidation in the mitochondrial matrix. The slowest step in this process (1 in Fig. 1.4) is the formation of acyl-carnitine required for transport into the matrix. Malonyl-CoA, an intermediate in fatty acid synthesis, inhibits step 1 at concentrations that prevail when synthesis is occurring. Thus β-oxidation is inhibited when fatty acid synthesis is active (Fig. 1.4). When synthesis is

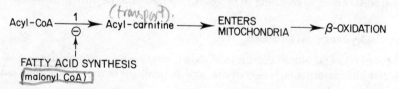

Fig. 1.4 Control of β-oxidation.

inactive, β-oxidation is limited by supply of fatty acyl-CoA and carnitine. Thus in muscle, where synthesis is of little importance, the rate of β-oxidation reflects the supply of fatty acid to the tissue which itself reflects lipolysis rates.

Ketone body metabolism

In man ketone bodies (acetoacetate and 3-hydroxybutyrate) are synthesized in liver when β-oxidation rates are elevated. Thus increased lipolysis is usually accompanied by ketonaemia. Ketogenesis from acetyl-CoA occurs when the rate of supply of acetyl-CoA (from β-oxidation) outstrips the capacity for its oxidation by the citric acid cycle. This process only occurs in liver because in this tissue there is (a) a limitation of citric acid cycle capacity and (b) the enzyme pathway for ketogenesis. The stoichiometry of acetoacetate synthesis and the kinetic properties of the enzymes of the pathway give a rate of acetoacetate synthesis that is proportional to the square of the rate of β-oxidation. In addition, the increased NADH/NAD ratio resulting from rapid β-oxidation in liver (which is partly responsible for decreased citric acid cycle capacity—see p. 10) causes a significant proportion of acetoacetate to be reduced to 3-hydroxybutyrate. Ketone body utilization (Fig. 1.5) occurs rapidly in extrahepatic tissues such as heart and

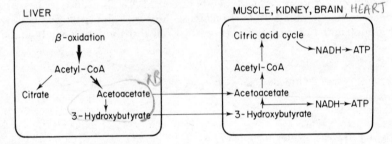

Fig. 1.5   Ketone body mobilization.

skeletal muscle and kidney, the resulting acetyl-CoA being oxidized without limitation in these tissues. Utilization of ketone bodies by the liver does not occur because this tissue lacks the enzyme 3 oxo-acid-CoA transferase which catalyses the transfer of Coenzyme A from succinyl CoA to acetoacetate. In brain, provided that plasma concentrations of ketone bodies are sufficiently high to allow rapid uptake, acetoacetate and 3-hydroxybutyrate are significant fuels. Thus the production of ketone bodies by liver and their oxidation by extrahepatic tissues is dramatically stimulated by those hormonal changes resulting in increased lipolysis and hepatic β-oxidation.

Carbohydrate catabolism

As with fat catabolism this can be divided into two phases: mobilization of stored glucose units (glycogenolysis) and breakdown of the glucose molecule (glycolysis).

Glycogenolysis

Glycogen comprises most of the body's stores of glucose and these glycogen stores are found primarily in liver and muscle. Their mobilization is controlled by the activity of glycogen phosphorylase. Rapid mobilization of glucose units in liver and muscle occurs as a result of raised adrenaline or decreased insulin concentration or raised glucagon levels (liver only) (Table 1.2). While the molecular details of these events are not yet clear in the

Table 1.2 Consequences of glycogenolysis in liver and muscle

Hormone change	Tissue	Glycogen to glucose	Glycogen to pyruvate
Insulin ↓ Adrenaline ↑ Glucagon ↑	Liver	+ + +	− (by glucagon)
Insulin ↓ Adrenaline ↑	Muscle	Not occur	+ + +

case of the insulin effect, the consequences of raised plasma adrenaline on the activity of glycogen phosphorylase in muscle have been described in detail and similar events occur with glucagon in liver. In both these cases a small increase in the plasma concentration of the hormones results in increased binding to tissue plasma membrane receptors initiating an increased rate of synthesis of cAMP. The elevated concentration of this intracellular messenger stimulates protein kinase activity which initiates an enzyme cascade involving specific kinases and phosphatases resulting in the net phosphorylation of phosphorylase **b** to the active **a** form (Fig. 1.6). In liver the effects of adrenaline (and angiotensin II and vasopressin) are not mediated by cAMP but by an increase in the concentration of free Ca^{2+}. This directly activates phosphorylase **b** kinase. Similarly in muscle an increase in free Ca^{2+} concentration (the result of neural action) can independently initiate the cascade resulting in stimulated glycogen breakdown. Additionally, in both tissues, the simultaneous inactivation of glycogen synthesis minimizes the

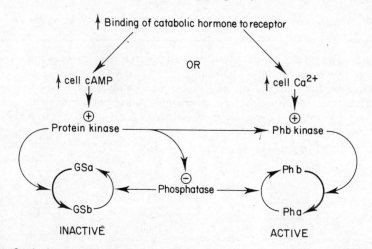

Fig. 1.6 Activation of phosphorylase (Ph) and inhibition of glycogen synthase (GS).

wasteful cycling of glucose units (Fig. 1.6). Phosphorylase is itself an allosteric enzyme showing susceptibility to a variety of physiological effectors (Table 1.3). Phosphorylation confers activity by stabilizing the active conformation of the enzyme even in the absence of an allosteric activator and only glucose (the product) is a significant inhibitor of the phosphorylated form.

Table 1.3 Physiological effectors of phosphorylase

Phosphorylase form and activity	Inhibitor	Activator	Tissue where effect is important
b Inactive without AMP	ATP Glucose-6-P	AMP	Muscle
a Active without AMP	Glucose	—	Liver

Glycolysis

Breakdown of glucose units to pyruvate is a pathway present in all tissues and can be used both for energy generation (exercising muscle) and for lipid synthesis from glucose units (liver and adipose tissue). When catabolic conditions prevail glycolysis is active in those tissues (muscle, brain, red cells but not liver) which derive a significant proportion of their energy requirements from glucose. Here the substrate is either derived from endogenous glycogen or from blood glucose derived from liver glycogen. In the case of adipose tissue and resting muscle the entry of glucose to the cell is insulin requiring (Table 1.4) but in working muscle glucose entry is less

Table 1.4 Effect of insulin on glucose transport across plasma membranes

Tissue	Stimulation by insulin
Liver	None
Brain	None
Muscle	+ + + but less in heavy exercise
Adipose	+ + +

dependent on insulin so that glycolysis can proceed from exogenous glucose in exercise even in catabolic conditions.

In muscle, brain and blood cells, glycolysis is controlled by energy demands mediated through the allosteric effectors of phosphofructokinase (Fig. 1.7). A sufficient supply of energy elevates ATP in relation to AMP

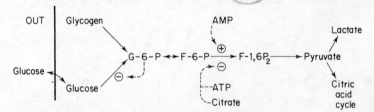

Fig. 1.7 Glycolysis in extrahepatic tissues.

which inhibits phosphofructokinase (PFK). In addition the rise in ATP concentration also slows the citric acid cycle (see later) resulting in raised cytosolic citrate. These changes inhibit PFK and the effect feeds back to hexokinase via elevated glucose-6-phosphate thus decreasing the rate of glucose entry to the pathway.

In liver raised glucagon inhibits glycolysis as a result of elevating cAMP concentrations which activates protein kinase. Two events now follow:

1. Pyruvate kinase is phosphorylated and in this form is inhibited by the prevailing PEP concentrations.
2. The level of fructose-2, 6 bisphosphate (F-2,6P$_2$) is decreased.

In liver glycolysis is regulated by F-2,6P$_2$ which is a very potent activator of phosphofructokinase antagonizing the inhibition by ATP and citrate. Decreased F-2,6P$_2$ thus results in lowered activity of phosphofructokinase. Hepatic glycolysis is therefore inhibited at two points by elevated glucagon (Fig. 1.8).

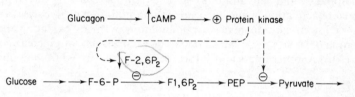

Fig. 1.8 Hepatic glycolysis.

Pyruvate oxidation

Oxidation of pyruvate to acetyl-CoA is irreversible and represents a loss to body carbohydrate reserves because animal cells lack the capacity for synthesis of glucose from acetyl-CoA. Regulation of this step is therefore essential. Pyruvate dehydrogenase exists in a phosphorylated (inactive) and dephosphorylated (active) form. These are interconvertible by a phosphatase and kinase (Fig. 1.9). The system does not respond to changes in cAMP but insulin is found to increase the amount of the active enzyme by stimulating the phosphatase. Additionally a raised cell Ca^{2+} will also activate the

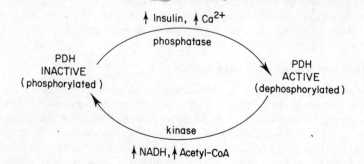

Fig. 1.9 Pyruvate dehydrogenase control.

phosphatase resulting in increased pyruvate dehydrogenase activity. The kinase is activated by elevated acetyl-CoA and NADH concentrations which therefore inhibit pyruvate oxidation. Therefore, except in exercising muscle where Ca^{2+} is elevated, pyruvate oxidation is inhibited by the decreased insulin of the catabolic state and is also inhibited when another source of acetyl-CoA (e.g. from β-oxidation) is available or when the cell redox state rises.

Gluconeogenesis

This occurs only in liver and kidney and, although it involves synthesis and is generally considered to be anabolic, it is in practice a response to stress situations, being part of the process of glucose production from protein catabolism (see next section). The pathway is stimulated by raised plasma glucagon and glucocorticoid, and lowered insulin concentrations. The former acts by removing fructose -2,6 bisphosphate an inhibitor of fructose 1,6 bisphosphatase and activator of PFK. The result of removing this compound is therefore activation of gluconeogenesis and inhibition of glycolysis. In addition, lowered insulin concentration inhibits pyruvate oxidation allowing utilization of lactate, pyruvate and alanine as substrates for gluconeogenesis (Fig. 1.10). Another important substrate is glycerol derived from lipolysis in

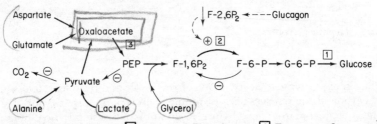

Fig. 1.10   Gluconeogenesis. [1] Glucose-6-Phosphatase; [2] Fructose 1:6 bisphosphatase; [3] Phosphoenolpyruvate carboxykinase.

adipose tissue. Chronic changes induced by glucagon and glucocorticoids include increased amounts of enzymes 1,2 and 3 (Fig. 1.10). Ultimately the pathway can be limited by substrate supply since utilization of all substrates can be inhibited by high redox states ($NADH/NAD^+$ ratios). Such a situation occurs upon excessive alcohol ingestion where the metabolism of ethanol elevates $NADH/NAD^+$ and inhibits gluconeogenesis.

Protein and amino acid catabolism

In an average adult man of approximately 70 kg body weight about 400 g of protein is broken down per day. This is part of the continual turnover of body proteins and is balanced by an equal rate of synthesis. Even in catabolic states only a fraction of this rate of protein breakdown to amino acid is ever used to fuel energy metabolism. While the mechanism of control of protein breakdown is unknown the process is stimulated in liver by raised plasma glucagon and in muscle and liver by elevated glucocorticoids. These effects are offset by the inhibition of degradation by raised insulin. The balance of these hormones thus determines the net rate of protein degradation to amino acids (Fig. 1.11).

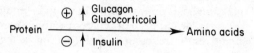

Fig. 1.11 Protein degradation.

Amino acid catabolism

Breakdown of amino acids involves their initial transamination followed by elimination of the α-amino group as urea and the catabolism of the remaining C-skeleton (Fig. 1.12). Acute regulation of these processes is by the

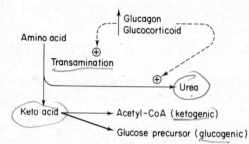

Fig. 1.12 Amino acid catabolism.

concentration of substrate and is therefore ultimately dependent on the net rate of protein breakdown. Glucagon and glucocorticoids increase amino acid catabolism chronically by increasing the amounts of the enzymes concerned. Glucagon exerts an acute stimulation on the uptake (and subsequent metabolism) of circulating alanine by the liver and this is important in catabolism of muscle protein-derived amino-acids. Because liver is the only tissue capable of synthesizing urea the α-amino groups derived from transaminated muscle amino acids have to be transported to liver. This is achieved by the glucose alanine cycle (Fig. 1.13). The control of the breakdown of the C-skeleton of amino acids depends on the nature of the

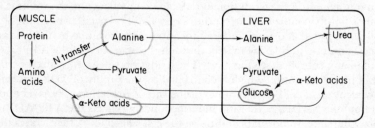

Fig. 1.13 Glucose alanine cycle.

α-ketoacid produced. Most enter the citric acid cycle or glycolysis or gluconeogenesis (glucogenic amino acids). Those derived from the essential branched chain amino acids (valine, isoleucine and leucine) are first decarboxylated by an enzyme complex similar to pyruvate dehydrogenase. The activity of this complex is under control by a kinase and phosphatase but further details are not known at present. Under catabolic conditions the metabolism of leucine results in ketone body formation (ketogenic amino acid).

Control of the citric acid cycle and oxidative phosphorylation

In mammalian tissues the major limitation of this pathway is redox state particularly the $NADH/NAD^+$ ratio. This ratio exerts its control by mass action and product inhibition on the dehydrogenases of the cycle (Fig. 1.14).

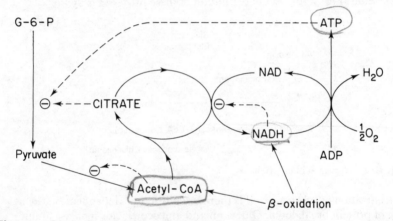

Fig. 1.14   Limitation of citric acid cycle rate by ATP via NADH.

In addition a high rate of acetyl-CoA input (derived from glycolysis and β-oxidation) to the cycle is reflected by an elevated citrate level which can overflow into the cytosol, thereby inhibiting glycolysis and reducing substrate supply to the cycle. This results in the sparing of carbohydrate at the expense of fat. In liver, the low maximal activity of citrate synthase limits the capacity of the cycle to the extent that acetyl-CoA produced at high rates (e.g. from β-oxidation) overflow into ketone body production.

In mitochondria the oxidation of reducing equivalents by the respiratory chain is tightly coupled to the synthesis of ATP. This occurs via a flow of protons extruded across the inner mitochondrial membrane by the oxidative process and re-entering the matrix through the operation of the ATP synthesizing complex (see Fig. 6.2). The oxidation rate is influenced by the rate of phosphorylation which is controlled by the supply of ADP and the concentration of ATP (the product). The rate of oxidation of NADH and therefore the NADH/NAD ratio in mitochondria reflects the ATP/ADP ratio. Therefore, in normal conditions, the cell's need for ATP dictates the level of mitochondrial NADH and this ultimately controls the dehydrogenases of the citric acid cycle. In brown adipose tissue the link between oxidation and phosphorylation is disrupted by the activity of a protein located in the inner membrane of the mitochondria (Chapter 6). This protein allows a short circuit in the normal flow of protons thus allowing re-entry of protons without ATP synthesis. This uncoupling of phosphorylation and oxidation results in high rates of heat generation due to unrestrained oxidation rates and high citric acid cycle activity.

Anabolism

The hormonal milieu characteristic of this state is one of elevated concentrations of insulin in relation to glucagon, catecholamines and glucocorticoids. This is seen in the immediate post prandial stage where insulin is the dominant hormone following stimulation of its release from β-cells by glucose, amino acids and possibly gastric inhibitory peptide. It is under the influence of this hormone that the synthesis of energy stores (glycogen, triglyceride) and the synthesis of protein takes place. It will be apparent that although insulin exerts major effects on metabolism in this state, the exact mechanism of its action is not understood. All that is known is that the initial event involves binding of insulin to a specific plasma membrane receptor.

Glycogen synthesis

The greatest fluctuations in glycogen concentrations occur in liver and in this tissue glycogen attains its highest concentration. This is because, after digestion, the hepatic portal vein carries large concentrations of glucose (often more than 10 mM) to the liver and, simultaneously, this organ receives newly secreted insulin by the same route. The combination of high insulin and glucose results in rapid glycogen synthesis, primarily due to rapid activation of glycogen synthase. This enzyme, inactive in the phosphorylated form, is activated by the same phosphatase that acts upon phosphorylase **a**. Thus the phosphatase activates glycogen synthesis and inhibits glycogenolysis. In liver this phosphatase is mainly bound to phosphorylase **a** forming an inactive complex. Glucose at concentrations greater than 5 mM binds to phosphorylase **a** (the glucose receptor in liver) changing the shape of the **a** form so that it is now acted upon by the phosphatase. As phosphorylase **a** is converted to the inactive **b** form the phosphatase is released and is now able to activate glycogen synthase. Thus free glucose in liver stimulates its own conversion into glycogen (Fig. 1.15). The role of insulin in this process, although essential, is unknown. In addition to this effect, the combination of high insulin and glucose maintains the synthesis of hepatic glucokinase ensuring a continued net flux of glucose into liver glycogen. In muscle the stimulation of glycogen synthesis by insulin also occurs via a cAMP independent process which results in the activation of the phosphatase common to the phosphorylase-synthase system. The response of glycogen synthesis in muscle to insulin requires lower concentrations than are needed

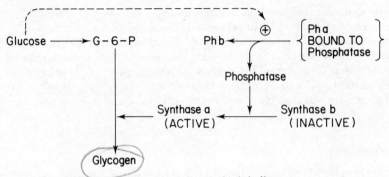

Fig. 1.15   Glucose stimulation of glycogen synthesis in liver.

for synthesis of glycogen in liver. In muscle (as in adipose tissue) insulin also stimulates the rate of glucose transport across the plasma membrane.

Lipogenesis

A major function of lipogenesis is to store (as triglyceride) the chemical energy of ingested foodstuffs when in excess of the immediate requirements of the organism. Additional functions however involve the assembly of phospholipids and sterols, both essential components of eukaryotic cell membranes.

Control of fatty acid synthesis

The rate limiting enzyme of the pathway is acetyl-CoA carboxylase which is the main target for the acute stimulation of the pathway by insulin and inhibition by glucagon (in liver) and adrenaline (in adipose tissue). Acetyl-CoA carboxylase is subject to control by covalent modification (phosphorylation) and allosteric effectors (Fig. 1.16). Phosphorylation of the

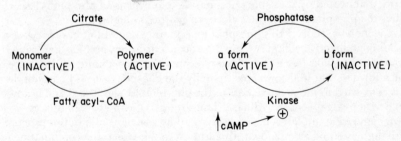

Fig. 1.16   Control of acetyl-CoA carboxylase activity.

enzyme by the cAMP-stimulated protein kinase increases its sensitivity to the inhibitory long chain acyl-CoA while decreasing its sensitivity to activation by citrate. These modes of control are not necessarily mutually exclusive and both act to decrease the activity of the enzyme. Acute inhibition of acetyl-

CoA carboxylase by glucagon and adrenaline in liver and adipocytes occurs via a cAMP dependent process but the rapid activation of the enzyme by insulin which also involves covalent modification, does not require cAMP.

In liver the preferred precursors for fatty acid synthesis are endogenous glycogen-derived glucose, lactate and blood glucose. The source of acetyl-CoA for this process is pyruvate and raised insulin concentrations cause the maximum activation of pyruvate dehydrogenase (see p. 7). This allows continued citrate synthesis from pyruvate-derived acetyl-CoA and hence activation of acetyl-CoA carboxylase. Pyruvate supply is ensured by the raised insulin and lowered glucagon levels which result in elevated fructose-6-phosphate and fructose 2,6 bisphosphate concentrations. These activate phosphofructokinase even in the presence of cytosolic citrate (see p. 7) resulting in active glycolysis. Control of the whole process is summarized in Fig. 1.17.

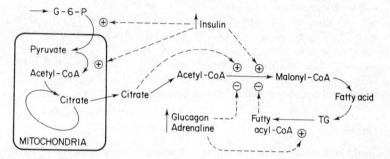

Fig. 1.17 Control of fatty acid synthesis.

It should be noted that the inhibitory effect of malonyl-CoA on β-oxidation prevents this pathway from supplying acetyl-CoA and also prevents significant futile cycling (Chapter 6).

In addition to its acute effects, raised insulin causes chronic stimulation via an increased amount of acetyl-CoA carboxylase and many of the cytosolic enzymes involved in glycolysis and fatty acid synthesis.

Control of triglyceride synthesis

The rate of this pathway in both liver and adipocytes appears to depend mainly on substrate supply, in particular fatty acyl-CoA. Thus triglyceride synthesis can be elevated under any condition in which fatty acid concentrations are raised in the tissue. In the fed state the raised insulin and lowered glucagon and adrenaline ensures that triglyceride breakdown is minimal so that fatty acid is supplied from endogenous synthesis or from the diet. Chronic control of triglyceride synthesis is exerted by phosphatidate phosphatase, the enzyme located at the branch point of triglyceride and phospholipid synthesis (Fig. 1.18). The activity of this enzyme is increased by elevated glucocorticoids but it is always sufficiently active for basal triglyceride synthesis.

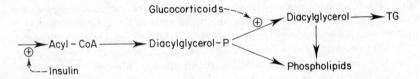

Fig. 1.18   Control of triglyceride (TG) synthesis.

Control of sterol synthesis

HMG-CoA reductase, the rate limiting enzyme of the pathway, is subject to a variety of controls. Acute regulation is by covalent modification involving two cycles of phosphorylation and dephosphorylation (see Chapter 8). The phosphorylated form is inactive and is increased by glucagon, whereas insulin causes dephosphorylation and activation. These hormones also exert chronic control over the total amount of the enzyme. In diabetes or in starvation the amount is greatly reduced and this occurs rapidly due to the short half life (2 h) of the enzyme. The amount of reductase is also decreased by accumulation of cellular cholesterol. These effects result in strict dietary control of sterol synthesis, inhibition of the pathway under catabolic conditions and activation when insulin concentrations are elevated.

Lipid export from liver

The pathways of sterol and triglyceride synthesis converge in the assembly of very low density lipoprotein (VLDL) in liver. Synthesis and secretion of this particle is stimulated by insulin and to some extent by raised glucocorticoids. The effect of both these hormones is at least partly due to increased substrate supply.

The fate of VLDL triglyceride depends on the hormonal state (Fig. 1.19). At elevated insulin concentrations the high activity of adipose tissue lipoprotein lipase ensures VLDL metabolism by that tissue resulting in the increased peripheral triglyceride stores. Under stress conditions when glucocorticoids are elevated and insulin is low the VLDL is preferentially

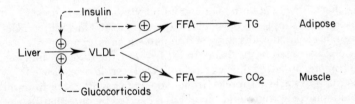

Fig. 1.19   Lipid export from liver.

metabolized by muscle. The lipoprotein lipase of heart and skeletal muscle is increased in activity by 'stress' hormones while the enzyme of adipose tissue is low in activity under these conditions. Metabolism of the triglyceride-derived fatty acids in muscle is by β-oxidation.

The cholesterol ester component of the VLDL remnant is taken up by liver or extrahepatic tissues as described in Chapter 8. This process is not under any hormonal control, being regulated by the cholesterol content of the tissue is question.

Protein synthesis and turnover

The 70 kg man supports a protein synthesis rate in excess of 400 g per day as part of normal protein turnover. The dietary input of amino acids is around 70 g per day and is clearly small compared to the supply created by turnover. The hepatic portal vein delivers the dietary input to the liver where all except

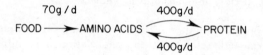

Fig. 1.20   Protein synthesis.

branched chain amino acids are metabolized to protein or catabolized. After a high protein meal the elevated amino acid level stimulates glucagon release from pancreatic α-cells in addition to the normal stimulation of insulin release from β-cells. The increased glucagon stimulates hepatic extraction of amino acids and allows sufficient gluconeogenesis to prevent insulin stimulated hypoglycaemia. Therefore even in the fed state some conversion of amino acid to glucose occurs. Branched chain amino acid uptake by muscle is stimulated by insulin and in muscle they are used for protein synthesis or transaminated and catabolized.

While the steps of protein synthesis in eukaryotic cells are now well documented the mechanism by which hormones control the process is not yet clear. In the fed state protein synthesis is stimulated by raised insulin and by growth hormone which exerts its anabolic effects in the presence of high insulin concentrations.

In eukaryotes (as in simpler organisms) protein synthesis is an integral part of gene expression and is controlled to a large extent by transcription.

$$DNA \xrightarrow{\text{transcription}} RNA \xrightarrow{\text{translation}} protein$$

This can result in a general increase in protein synthesis (translation) through the provision of more t-RNA, ribosomes, and m-RNA or can specifically provide an increase in just one m-RNA species. The process is relatively slow and can be described as chronic in nature. Both insulin and growth hormone stimulate transcription in muscle and liver. By analogy with the mechanism of action of the polypeptide growth factors (nerve and epidermal) the process may involve internalization of the polypeptide-plasma-membrane-receptor complex and subsequent delivery to the nucleus after prior fusion and processing in lysosomes.

The acute effects of insulin on protein synthesis are due to two actions. Firstly insulin stimulates amino acid transport across muscle cell membrane thus providing an increased supply of substrate for amino acyl-t-RNA formation. Secondly insulin stimulates the initiation reaction of protein synthesis in liver and muscle resulting in increased polysome number and increased translation of RNA into protein (Fig. 1.21). In the case of globin

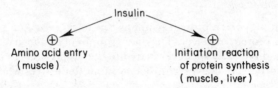

Fig. 1.21   Acute effects of insulin on protein synthesis.

synthesis the process of initiation is controlled by a cAMP-stimulated protein kinase-initiated cascade resulting in phosphorylation and inhibition of an essential initiation factor (protein) eIF-2. Whether this process is general and whether it is applicable to the acute action of insulin remains to be discovered.

2

Starvation

Starvation or fasting is defined as the state of deprivation of food. In this state the length of survival depends not only on the amount and nature of the reserves of food stored in the body but also on the metabolic adaptations that control the use of these reserves. The body fuel reserves of the 'average' man are given in Table 2.1 and it is clear that even in the lean average individual

Table 2.1 Fuel reserves in the average 70 kg man

Fuel	Tissue	Energy
Fat (triglyceride)	Adipose tissue	100 000 kcal
Carbohydrate (glycogen)	Liver	200 kcal
	Muscle	400 kcal
(glucose)	Body fluids	40 kcal
Protein	Muscle	25 000 kcal
		(<8 000 kcal available)

fat accounts for the majority of these reserves. Protein (chiefly muscle protein) is included but it should be noted that loss of even one-third of body protein is probably not compatible with survival. Assuming that the mechanism exists for avoiding consumption of essential protein we can calculate that with a basal energy expenditure of 1 700 kcal/day our average man should be able to survive starvation for at least 2 months (assuming an adequate supply of water). In fact a variety of studies with obese volunteers have shown that, provided the subject is initially upholstered with enough fat, he or she can easily survive a fast of 6 months or more under medical supervision. It is clear then that starvation must be accompanied by metabolic controls that switch fuel consumption to the burning of fat and minimise the consumption of carbohydrate and essential protein.

Before discussing the hormonal and metabolic adaptations that occur in starvation it is important to consider the major energy consuming tissues of the body (Table 2.2). Brain alone of these is incapable of deriving energy from oxidation of fatty acids and since the preferred fuel for adult brain is glucose the successful adaptation to starvation must involve glucose homoeostasis as a priority.

The major hormonal response to starvation is a fall in concentration of

Table 2.2 Tissue fuel consumption in the 70 kg man (resting)

Tissue	Wet weight (kg)	O_2 consumption (ml/min.)	Fuel*
Skeletal muscle	20–30	70	G,K,F
Adipose	9–13	Small	G,F
Gastrointestinal tract	2.6	58	G,K,F
Blood, etc.	5.5	Small	G
Liver	1.7	75	G,F
Brain	1.5	46	G,K
Lung	1.0	12	G,K,F
Heart	0.3	27	G,K,F
Kidney	0.3	16	G,K,F

* G = glucose, K = ketone bodies, F = fatty acids, not in order of preference.

plasma insulin and rise in plasma glucagon concentration both triggered by an initial drop in blood glucose (Fig. 2.1). At least in the case of therapeutic starvation the concentrations of other relevant hormones such as growth hormone, glucocorticoids and catecholamines do not show any consistent change from normal. The immediate result of these hormonal changes is a switch of body metabolism into a catabolic mode causing liver glycogenolysis, gluconeogenesis, adipose tissue lipolysis and increased muscle proteolysis (Table A.2). Work by Cahill, Owen, Felig and others has established that the response to starvation follows a biphasic mode. This can be seen in the changes in blood parameters in Fig. 2.1. The first phase, occurring over 3–7 days is marked by dramatic changes in insulin and glucagon concentrations and a drop in blood glucose level of around 1 mM. The second phase, extending from 7 days onwards is characterized by an almost steady state in these parameters. Felig has described these two phases in terms of the adaptations made to allow survival. The initial response to starvation is concerned with the maintenance of glucose production to meet the needs of the brain (gluconeogenic phase). The later phase is one of protein conservation in which the derivation of glucose from protein breakdown is minimized and even brain metabolism switches away from glucose as the main fuel.

Gluconeogenic phase

In this stage the supply of glucose for the brain is maintained by two mechanisms:

1. Glucose mobilization from hepatic glycogen stores accompanied by increased liver gluconeogenesis.
2. Decreased glucose oxidation by muscle and other tissues capable of using alternative fuels.

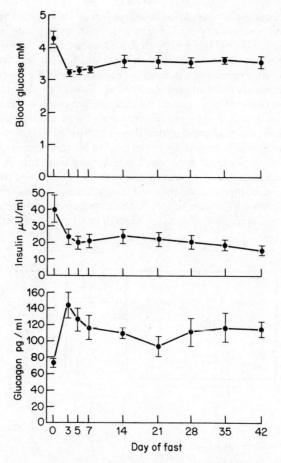

Fig. 2.1 Blood glucose, serum insulin and plasma glucagon response to prolonged starvation. The subjects studied were seven obese volunteers. Values are mean ± SEM. (Reproduced from Marliss et al. (1970). *J. Clin. Invest.*, **49**, 2256, by copyright permission of The American Society for Clinical Investigation.)

Increased glucose mobilization and synthesis

The fall in blood glucose concentration occurring early in starvation causes a large fall in plasma insulin concentration and a subsequent rise in plasma glucagon concentration (Fig. 2.1). As in a normal overnight starvation the initial response to these changes is the mobilization of liver glycogen stores (Fig. 1.6). But these stores are limited in amount and even during overnight starvation the high rate of brain metabolism (420 kcal/day; 120 g of glucose/day) requires that 25 per cent of glucose production is provided by hepatic gluconeogenesis. At this rate of gluconeogenesis the glucose precursors are mainly lactate and pyruvate plus a small contribution from glycerol released during lipolysis. As the period of starvation lengthens the continuing increase in glucagon/insulin ratio results in mobilization of fatty acids and increased hepatic β-oxidation of fatty acid (Fig. 1.2) inhibiting pyruvate oxidation (Fig. 1.9) and providing the energy to drive increased gluconeogenesis. Furthermore the continuing decrease in blood insulin concentration allows increased protein degradation in muscle (Fig. 1.11) leading to a considerable rise in net amino acid output (primarily as alanine). The elevated concentration of blood glucagon stimulates the hepatic extraction of alanine from the circulation and thus provides increased flow of substrate to sustain the already stimulated gluconeogenic flux. Thus by 36 h starvation, gluconeogenesis is now providing 75 per cent of hepatic glucose production and more than 50 per cent of this glucose is derived from muscle protein breakdown via alanine. In starvation the normal operation of the glucose alanine cycle (Chapter 1) is interrupted so that amino acids derived from protein breakdown in muscle supply both the pyruvate and the amino group for the synthesis of alanine (Fig. 2.2). Thus in early stages of starvation

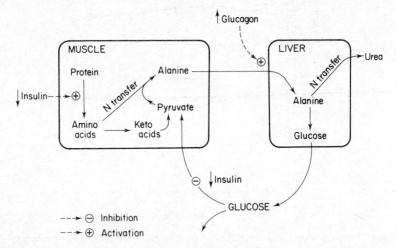

Fig. 2.2   Glucose-alanine interrelationships in starvation.

alanine formation and release correlates well with muscle protein degradation but not with muscle glucose utilization. Studies of metabolism of amino acids in muscle during starvation indicate that those most rapidly converted to pyruvate include the branched chain amino acids (except ketogenic leucine). These amino acids can make a net carbon contribution to C_4-intermediates of the citric acid cycle in muscle and can then produce pyruvate via phosphoenolpyruvate and phosphoenolpyruvate carboxykinase. The control of this interruption of the glucose alanine cycle during starvation is not clear but it must include the greatly reduced extraction of blood glucose by muscle resulting from decreased circulating insulin. It is worth noting that the elevated plasma glucagon does not cause mobilization of muscle glycogen glucose which therefore does not provide a source of pyruvate for alanine synthesis.

In summary, as a result of the increasing plasma glucagon concentration and decreasing insulin concentration early in starvation there is a rapid hepatic glycogenolysis together with and eventually replaced by glucose provision by hepatic gluconeogenesis from alanine derived from increased muscle proteolysis (Fig. 2.3).

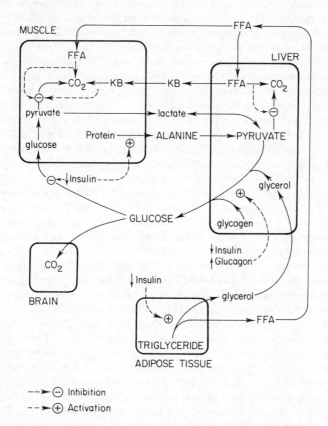

Fig. 2.3 Glucose sparing for use by brain in the early phase of starvation. KB = ketone bodies (acetoacetate, 3 hydroxy-butyrate). FFA = free fatty acids (long chain).

Decreased glucose oxidation

In order to allow hepatic glucose production to supply adequately the oxidative needs of brain metabolism there has to be a mechanism for sparing glucose oxidation by other tissues. This is achieved in two ways. Firstly, the rate of glucose entry to muscle and lung and adipose cells (an insulin dependent process) is diminished due to the fall in insulin and glucose concentrations. Secondly, the onset of starvation is accompanied by the provision of fatty acids and ketone bodies (acetoacetate and 3-hydroxybutyrate) as alternative fuels. With the exception of brain and the obligatorily glycolytic tissues such as red blood cells, kidney medulla, etc., body tissues do not use glucose as their sole oxidative fuel (Table 2.2).

Even within the period of an overnight fast the drop in plasma insulin concentration is sufficient to cause significant lipolysis in adipose tissue with release of long chain fatty acids into the circulation (Fig. 1.2). Liver responds to the resulting rise in glucagon/insulin ratio by increased β-oxidation of these fatty acids leading to significant ketogenesis (Fig. 1.5) and the rate of this latter process continues to increase in the early days of starvation. Plasma ketone body concentrations change more rapidly than fatty acid concentrations showing a more than 50-fold increase (to 0.6 mmol) in the first 2 days of starvation whereas fatty acid levels rise 2 to 3-fold only. Ketone bodies are a good fuel for a wide variety of tissues and their production by liver can be regarded as a way of exporting the excess 'ATP equivalents' produced by rapid β-oxidation in the liver to other tissues. Thus during the first phase of starvation ketone body production is matched by extrahepatic consumption and the excretion of excess in the urine (ketonuria) is absent.

Ketone bodies have some advantages as fuels for extrahepatic tissues (especially resting muscle) in starvation. There is no limit to their transport through body water to the sites of their oxidation in extrahepatic tissues since ketone bodies are freely water soluble. Unlike long chain fatty acids, whose low solubility in interstitial water may limit their use by resting muscle, ketone bodies would have free access to this tissue. Furthermore their transport into muscle is insulin independent (unlike glucose transport) and would not be restricted during starvation. Finally ketone bodies have an antilipolytic effect in normal individuals. The mechanism is not clear but it involves a stimulation of insulin release from pancreatic β-cells as well as a direct inhibition by ketone bodies of adipose tissue lipolysis. The result is that the rate of ketone body consumption can to some extent regulate their production. As well as providing an alternative to glucose, the metabolism of ketone bodies and fatty acids inhibits glucose oxidation in extrahepatic tissues. The increased degree of acetylation of coenzyme A caused by rapid oxidation of ketone bodies and fatty acids increases the proportion of the inactive (phosphorylated) form of pyruvate dehydrogenase (Fig. 1.9) thus preventing irreversible loss of glucose carbon. Any glycolytic breakdown of glucose would thus be channelled to lactate and can be converted to glucose again by hepatic gluconeogenesis. Thus, in starvation, the Cori cycle driven by fatty acid oxidation in liver is maintained by the glucose sparing actions of fatty acid and ketone body oxidation in muscle. These actions of fatty acids and ketone bodies, resulting in the sparing of glucose for brain metabolism during the early phase of starvation, are shown in Fig. 2.3.

Protein conservation phase

While this phase is characterized by an almost steady state hormonal milieu two metabolic changes take place which are essential to survival: 1. oxidation of ketone bodies by brain and 2. the inhibition of protein breakdown.

Ketone body oxidation by brain

During this second phase of starvation both urinary nitrogen excretion and plasma alanine concentration drop progressively with time indicating a reduction in the rate of gluconeogenesis. Over a 5-week fasting period hepatic glucose output is reduced by more than 70 per cent and, although the

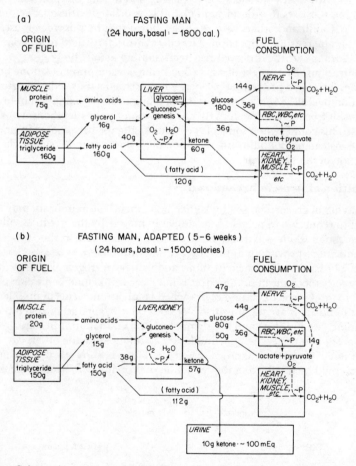

Fig. 2.4 Schematic representation of substrate metabolism in man after a short period of fasting (36 h) (a) and after a prolonged period of fasting (5 to 6 weeks) (b). (Reproduced from Reynold, A.C., Stauffacher, W. and Cahill, G. F. *The Metabolic Basis of Inherited Disease*. Ed. by Stanbury et al. McGraw Hill Book Company: New York.)

kidney cortex now carries out significant gluconeogenesis (equal to the output of liver), the total would not meet the brain's needs. The fact that blood glucose level remains unchanged indicates that brain metabolism has switched to another fuel. Owen, Cahill and co-workers have shown that over this period brain adapts to oxidize ketone bodies. The exact nature of the adaptation is uncertain; it may involve an increase in activity (induction) of ketone body metabolizing enzymes as well as the system for transporting ketone bodies into nerve cells. Note that neonatal and infant brain has a much higher capacity for metabolizing ketone bodies than unadapted adult brain and this probably reflects the ketones' higher rate of permeation into the cells of the young brain. Certainly brain metabolism of ketone bodies increases with their concentration in plasma and during this phase of starvation this rises to around 7 mmol and is associated with some ketonuria. Work by Cahill and others (Fig. 2.4) has shown that by this stage muscle derives an increasing proportion of its energy from fatty acid oxidation. This would account for the observed rise in circulating ketone body concentrations. By 4 weeks of starvation brain consumption of ketone bodies provides for 50–60 per cent of its energy requirements thus reducing glucose oxidation overall. Some further saving of glucose loss by oxidation in brain may result from inhibition of pyruvate oxidation by the metabolism of ketone bodies. This could switch some of the residual glucose breakdown in brain to lactate instead of CO_2 allowing retention of glucose carbon skeleton via the operation of the Cori cycle.

Inhibition of protein breakdown

The saving of glucose caused by ketone body metabolism in brain may be linked to reduction in protein breakdown in muscle by the rise in circulating ketone bodies. Both 3-hydroxy-butyrate and acetoacetate at the concentrations prevailing at this stage in starvation have been shown to reduce plasma alanine concentrations and urinary nitrogen excretion in man. The precise mechanism of this effect is not clear but ketone bodies have been found to inhibit the oxidation of branched chain amino acids in muscle. Since these amino acids are the precursors of both the carbon and nitrogen portions of alanine (see Fig. 2.2) and are themselves known to inhibit protein catabolism in muscle, their accumulation could mediate the observed inhibition of protein breakdown (Fig. 2.5). There is also little doubt that insulin could be involved in the reduction of protein catabolism by ketone

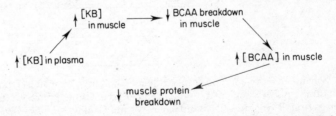

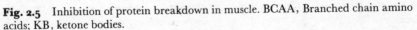

Fig. 2.5 Inhibition of protein breakdown in muscle. BCAA, Branched chain amino acids; KB, ketone bodies.

bodies since the hyperketonaemia of diabetic ketoacidosis (up to 20 mM) is associated with rapid rates of protein breakdown and urinary nitrogen excretion quite unlike the situation in long term starvation.

In summary (Fig. 2.6) the increased proportion of fatty acids oxidized by

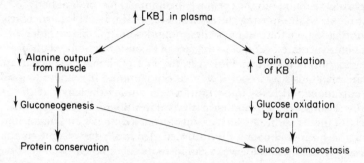

Fig. 2.6 Role of ketone bodies (KB) in protein conservation and glucose homoeostasis in prolonged starvation.

muscle in prolonged starvation allows a significant ketonaemia which has two results:

1. The sparing of glucose oxidation by brain due to cerebral ketone body metabolism.
2. The inhibition of protein breakdown in muscle allowing protein conservation and decreasing the rate of gluconeogenesis to maintain glucose homoeostasis.

Thus during prolonged starvation, body metabolism achieves a minimal level of glucose oxidation with considerable protein conservation while gearing itself to maximal use of fat as a fuel. As starvation proceeds the steady loss of weight due to fat metabolism allows additional energy saving by a decrease in daily energy expenditure needs.

Salt and water metabolism in starvation

Early starvation is marked by a rapid weight loss which is not due to energy expenditure but to transient Na^+ and water diuresis lasting 3 to 7 days. This is associated with the rapid rise in plasma glucagon concentrations (Fig. 2.1) and is thought to be due to the loss of liver glycogen occurring over this period. After this transient diuresis, further loss of Na^+ is very low reflecting the need for maintenance of body fluid volume. Urinary nitrogen loss in the early phase of starvation is accompanied by stoichiometric loss of K^+ (3 meq. per g of nitrogen) but this is very much reduced during the prolonged protein conservation phase of starvation. The decreased urinary nitrogen excretion is due to a virtual cessation of urea output. This drops from about 12 g/day early in starvation to less than 1 g/day after 5 weeks and serves to minimize water loss and reduce the need for water intake. The main excretory form of nitrogen during this phase is NH_4^+ produced by the kidney in part to maintain acid-base balance while ketone bodies (organic acids) are being excreted. This serves to retain Na^+ for maintenance of vascular volume.

The changes in metabolism during starvation illustrate the efficient integration of metabolism to achieve the minimal loss of vital body constituents while ensuring the maximal survival time. It is particularly interesting to note that many of these adaptations take place under metabolite mediated control in the face of a constant or only slightly changing hormonal milieu. However, this lack of change in concentration of insulin antagonists (glucocorticoids, catecholamines) in relation to insulin concentration is critically important in determining the length of the period of protein conservation and hence survival in starvation. This is shown clearly in those conditions such as uncontrolled diabetes and major injury where this hormonal balance is disturbed. Table 2.3 draws some comparisons between these states and serves as an introduction to their detailed discussion.

Table 2.3 A comparison of metabolic changes in starvation, uncontrolled diabetes mellitus and major injury

	Starvation	*Uncontrolled diabetes*	*Major injury*
Metabolic rate	↓	↑	↑
Energy source	Fat	Fat	Fat
Ketosis	+	+ + +	±
Gluconeogenesis	+ + + then +	+	+ + +
Nitrogen loss	+	+ + +	+ + +
Water Na^+	Initial loss	+ + +	Retention
K^+ loss	+	+ +	+ + +

Diabetes mellitus

Definition

Diabetes is a term applied to any condition in which there is excessive excretion of urine. Mellitus (latin—honeyed) reflects the finding that urine from patients with uncontrolled diabetes mellitus is sweet to taste. Diabetes mellitus can most simply be defined as a condition in which there is a marked and persistent hyperglycaemia.

Aetiology

Classically, two subclasses of the disease are described. Type I (juvenile onset; insulin dependent) is a condition of insulin deficiency whose aetiology is obscure and may represent a spectrum of disorders embracing HLA linked disease (B8, DW3, DW4) and viral infections. In contrast, the plasma concentration of insulin in type II (maturity onset; insulin independent) is often normal or even above normal. In this case there appears to be a resistance to insulin in peripheral tissues possibly as a result of a decrease in receptor number or affinity in the target cell.

Alterations in metabolism

Although the severe metabolic disturbances associated with uncontrolled type I diabetes are in part due to the (total) lack of the anabolic hormone (insulin) the unopposed actions of catabolic hormones (glucagon, cortisol) serve to exacerbate the situation and contribute significantly to the biochemical changes seen.

The result is a swing away from hormonally regulated metabolic homoeostasis in favour of catabolism. The major metabolic consequences of uncontrolled type I diabetes are listed in Table 3.1. The uptake of glucose from plasma by insulin-sensitive tissues such as skeletal muscle and adipose tissue is markedly reduced by the very low circulating insulin concentration and leads to a hyperglycaemic state as dietary glucose remains in the extracellular compartment. This is accompanied by a decrease in the

Table 3.1   Biochemical signs and their causes in diabetes mellitus

Biochemical signs	Cause
1. Hyperglycaemia	(i) Decreased uptake of glucose by peripheral tissues. (ii) Increased hepatic glycogen mobilization. (iii) Increased hepatic gluconeogenesis.
2. Glycosuria	Glucose load exceeds capacity for reabsorption in renal tubule.
3. Ketoacidosis	Increased β-oxidation of adipose tissue derived fatty acids in liver. Leads to raised hepatic acetyl CoA concentration and ketone body synthesis.
4. Ketonuria	Ketone load exceeds capacity for reabsorption in renal tubule.
5. Hyperlactataemia	Mobilization and metabolism of muscle glycogen to lactate: Lactate released as precursor of gluconeogenesis (Cori cycle).
6. Hyperlipidaemia	Free fatty acids derived from increased lipolysis in adipose tissue.
7. Hypertriglyceridaemia	Increased synthesis of triglyceride in liver and increased VLDL synthesis.
8. Hypovolaemia/ Hyperosmolarity	Excessive loss of body water as urine due to glucose acting as an osmotic diuretic.
9. Hyponatraemia	Loss of body sodium as a result of glucose-induced osmotic diuresis.

activities of the general anabolic pathways of lipogenesis and glycogenesis in liver, glycogenesis and protein synthesis in muscle and lipogenesis in adipose tissue (Table A.2). The increase in catabolic relative to anabolic hormone action promotes the mobilization of metabolic fuel stores. In skeletal muscle there is increased output of lactate from glycogenolysis and glycolytic metabolism of glycogen-derived glucose (Fig. 1.7) and also of glucogenic amino acids from increased proteolysis. The further metabolism of glucose (pyruvate) in muscle via the citric acid cycle is prevented by the reversible inhibition of pyruvate dehydrogenase by phosphorylation (Fig. 1.9).

The breakdown of stored triglyceride in adipose tissue is stimulated and there is a massive efflux of free fatty acids and glycerol-3 phosphate into the plasma. A high concentration of free fatty acids in the extracellular compartment inhibits glucose uptake by adipose tissue and skeletal muscle and assists in the maintenance of the hyperglycaemic state. In the liver further metabolism by β-oxidation of free fatty acids derived from adipose tissue triglyceride leads to the production of acetyl CoA and NADH with two major metabolic consequences:

1. The increase in concentration of NADH favours the production of glycerol-3 phosphate which in turn acts as acceptor of free fatty acids in the formation of triglyceride. These hepatically derived triglycerides are secreted as VLDL and create the hypertriglyceridaemia seen in uncontrolled diabetes.
2. Although some acetyl CoA is oxidized in the citric acid cycle this route

of disposal is soon saturated and the accumulation of acetyl CoA drives hepatic ketone body synthesis (Fig. 1.5). A ketoacidosis may develop and the smell of ketones can sometimes be detected on the breath of uncontrolled diabetics.

This shift from homoeostasis to enhanced catabolism promotes hepatic glycogenolysis and gluconeogenesis. The small amount of liver glycogen (Table 2.1) is rapidly exhausted while gluconeogenesis proceeds using the glucogenic amino acids and lactate provided by the catabolism of muscle. The combined actions of hepatic mobilization of glycogen and glucose synthesis contribute directly to the hyperglycaemic state.

Thus in biochemical terms the uncontrolled diabetic may be characterized by hyperglycaemia, hyperlipidaemia, hyperlactataemia from muscle glycogen breakdown, and ketoacidosis. Metabolically the diabetic state resembles that of the early stage of starvation with the body undergoing major changes in an attempt to supply its metabolic demands for fuel (Fig. 3.1). Despite the high extracellular glucose concentration the production and

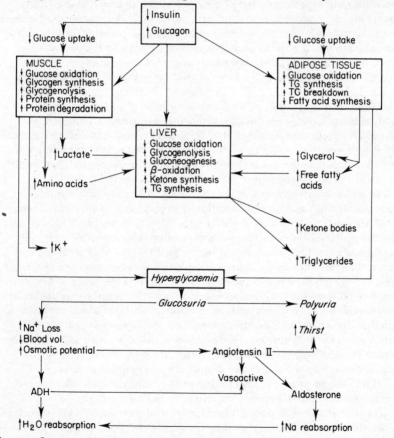

Fig. 3.1 Integrated biochemical and physiological relationships in diabetes mellitus. ADH = Antidiuretic hormone; TG = Triglyceride.

mobilization of glucose proceeds because of the inability of muscle and adipose tissue to take up this glucose. Such a condition has given rise to the aphorism 'starvation in the midst of plenty'. Obviously, dietary glucose contributes directly to hyperglycaemia but it is perhaps worth stressing that hepatic gluconeogenesis in the uncontrolled diabetic contributes significantly to the plasma glucose concentration and even in the absence of dietary glucose will give rise to hyperglycaemia.

Physiological and biochemical adaptations

These radical changes in metabolism produce profound physiological and endocrinological alterations in an attempt to achieve homoeostasis. The accumulation of acetoacetate, β-hydroxybutyrate and lactate create a metabolic acidosis and the fall in plasma pH acts as a powerful stimulator of respiration. Hyperventilation (Kussmaul breathing) is an involuntary respiratory attempt to raise the plasma pH by removal of dissolved CO_2. Plasma glucose concentration continues to rise until the glucose load exceeds the capacity of reabsorption in the renal tubules (9–10 mmol). At this stage some glucose remains in the renal tubule and appears in the urine (glycosuria). Similarly, the concentration of plasma ketones eventually exceeds the renal threshold for ketones, and ketonuria with consequential urinary acidification results. The presence of glucose in the renal tubule acts as an osmotic diuretic inhibiting the reabsorption of water and producing a highly diluted filtrate. This in turn alters the transtubular gradients of sodium and potassium ions such that these too are retained within the renal tubule and excreted. A highly dilute, possibly acidic urine containing glucose, sodium and potassium ions is therefore produced and polyuria (particularly nocturia) is a diagnostic feature of uncontrolled diabetes mellitus.

The major loss of body water creates a hypovolaemic, hyperosmolar extracellular fluid and increased sodium loss also leads to a hyponatraemic state. Although potassium is also excreted, this loss of the extracellular ion is offset by mobilization of intracellular potassium which stoichiometrically accompanies the efflux of amino acids released by lysis of skeletal muscle proteins. Further hormonal changes then occur as a consequence of the fall in blood volume and the rise in the osmotic potential of the plasma. Antidiuretic hormone (vasopressin) is released from the posterior pituitary as the atrial perfusion volume is reduced and the osmotic potential of blood perfusing the hypothalamus rises. This hormone promotes the increase in water reabsorption by the kidney collecting ducts in an attempt to maintain plasma volume (Chapter 9). It also has vasoconstrictor properties and acts to maintain systemic blood pressure despite the fall in blood volume.

A fall in the pressure of blood perfusing the kidney initiates the renin-angiotensin cascade (Chapter 9) resulting in the release of the mineralocorticosteroid, aldosterone, from the adrenal cortex. The release of aldosterone may also be increased by the direct effect of a reduced total plasma sodium. The combined actions of vasopressin and aldosterone will then serve to promote the movement of intracellular water into the extracellular space to try to maintain blood volume. Angiotensin II which is produced as an intermediate of the renin-aldosterone system (Chapter 9) and also as a consequence of increased vasomotor activity in response to hypovolaemia is a powerful vasoconstrictor and assists in the maintenance of systemic blood pressure. The hormone may also function as a neuropeptide, stimulating thirst receptors in the CNS and mediating the unsatiable thirst characteristic of uncontrolled diabetes. This is another reflex by which the body tries to maintain plasma volume.

Table 3.2 Clinical symptoms and their causes in diabetes mellitus

Symptoms	Cause
1. Polyuria (nocturia)	Retention of glucose in renal tubule as glucose load exceeds the absorptive capacity. Glucose acts as an osmotic diuretic causing the production of large volumes of urine.
2. Thirst	CNS driven response to dehydration. May be mediated by angiotensin produced in response to hypovolaemia.
3. Polyphagia	Hunger stimulated by non-utilization of dietary glucose.
4. Weight Loss	Increased catabolism of all metabolic fuel stores— muscle glycogen and protein and adipose tissue triglyceride.
5. Tiredness	Muscular weakness due to (i) proteolysis and mobilization of muscle protein (ii) reduced availability of metabolic substrate (glucose).
6. Blurred vision	Systemic dehydration of the lens, aqueous and vitreous humor reducing visual acuity.
7. Vomiting	CNS driven response to ketones stimulating the area postrema in the floor of the fourth ventricle.
8. Hyperventilation (Kussmaul breathing)	Respiratory compensation to metabolic acidosis (raised lactate and keto acids in plasma).
9. Itching	

Treatment

The only treatment for type I diabetes (insulin dependent) is daily, usually subcutaneous, administration of insulin; failure to do this is fatal. The less severe type II diabetes is treated either by diet, in an attempt to reduce insulin resistance, or by oral hypoglycaemic agents such as the biguanides or sulphonylureas, which serve to potentiate the activity of endogenous insulin.

Complications of diabetes mellitus

Even though the use of insulin has greatly reduced the deaths from type I diabetes there is still considerable mortality associated with the disease. For example, recent estimates suggest that the complications of diabetes may account for some 2–5 per cent of the total mortality in the United States. Probably many of the complications arise from poor control of the disease where plasma glucose is maintained at concentrations higher than are physiologically normal. It is postulated that persistent hyperglycaemia may result in non-specific protein glycosylation and lead to some of the common diabetic complications such as renal failure, peripheral vascular disease, retinopathies, blindness and peripheral neuropathies. Long standing diabetics are also prone to recurrent infection possibly due to non-specific immunodeficiency since a reduction in the efficiency of intracellular pathogen killing in polymorphogranulocytes has been found in such patients.

A more acute and life threatening complication of 'treated' diabetics is hypoglycaemia as a result of insulin overdose or of an inadequate carbohydrate intake. The symptoms of hypoglycaemia include sweating, tachycardia, hunger, mental confusion, paraesthesia, diplopia and coma (Table 3.2). The immediate treatment is administration of glucose either orally or intravenously.

4

Trauma

Early studies into the metabolic effects of injury were often hampered by the inability of the patient to survive the treatment of the initial shock phase. However improved nursing care has brought some understanding of the more chronic metabolic changes associated with trauma. Common features of major illness or injury (such as fatigue and weight loss) are easily noticed. For instance a 6 per cent weight loss may result from uncomplicated surgery while weight loss may be as much as 30 per cent following multiple fractures. These losses after trauma occur much faster than during starvation. A major contribution to the understanding of the metabolic changes after injury was made by Cuthbertson who described distinct stages in the response; an immediate shock or ebb phase of about 24 hours when cellular activity is depressed followed by a recovery or flow phase of hypermetabolism which may last for weeks. Complete recovery is achieved after a further restorative anabolic phase as lean body mass lost in the ebb phase is replaced.

The initial shock phase

It is well known in the animal kingdom that the central nervous system can prepare for the flight or fight situation facing an animal under threat. Even without injury this involves a release of adrenaline which in turn gives rise to an increase in blood pressure and heart rate and mobilization of glycogen from liver and muscle and triglyceride from adipose tissue. Such changes of the defence reaction are also seen in patients about to undergo surgery even before administration of the anaesthetic. The injury or insult itself then sets off a barrage of stimuli focussed mainly on the hypothalamus and hindbrain which releases a number of hormone releasing factors. These in turn act on the pituitary and cause the release of ACTH, prolactin, growth hormone, antidiuretic hormone and oxytocin. The role of some of these hormones in the injury response is not understood.

Thus metabolism in the initial shock or ebb phase is characteristic of a stress response and the immediate changes are due to a massive sympathetic response leading to the release of catecholamines. The decreased cellular vitality of this phase is often associated with loss of blood or plasma from the wound, and with a decrease in oxygen supply to peripheral tissues as the body seeks to conserve blood flow for vital organs. Although there is a decreased (resting) energy expenditure at this time the massive release of adrenaline causes, both directly and indirectly, a general mobilization of metabolizable substrates (Table 2.4). Serum concentrations of glucose and lactate (from liver and muscle) and free fatty acids (from adipose tissue) are raised. The release of adrenaline is also sufficient to inhibit insulin secretion by β-cells and stimulate glucagon secretion by the α-cells of the pancreas (Fig. 4.1). Thus at a time when the plasma glucose concentration rises,

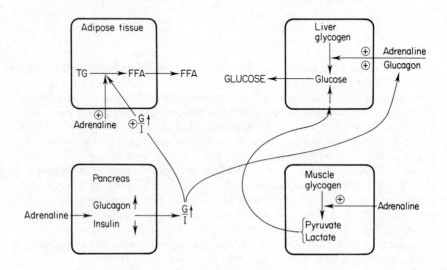

Fig. 4.1   Hormonal and metabolic changes during the ebb phase.

clearance of glucose by insulin-sensitive peripheral tissues, particularly muscle, is severely reduced due to an insulin lack. A glucose tolerance test performed 6 hours after severe trauma shows none only a slight insulin response. The raised fatty acid concentration and the release of growth hormone and cortisol, both insulin antagonists, also contribute to insulin resistance in the early stages after injury. Consequently there is an increased utilization of fatty acid as respiratory substrate and increased ketogenesis.

The hypermetabolic phase

The short period of depressed metabolism is followed by a hypermetabolic flow phase which may last for many weeks despite visual healing of wounds. This stage is characterized by increases in heat production, resting metabolic expenditure (RME), respiration and pulse rate, increases which are accentuated in burned patients where there is often considerable evaporative heat loss. Thus a healthy individual at rest in bed consumes approximately 25 kcal/kg/daily and increases this by about 20 per cent if allowed to walk freely in the ward. In order to maintain zero energy balance a food intake 20–30 per cent greater than the measured metabolic expenditure is required since such an individual utilizes food inefficiently. After minor surgery RME is increased by about 10 per cent; after multiple fractures by 20 per cent. This may be increased by 50 per cent on infection such as in peritonitis and even by as much as 100 per cent with major burns (Table 4.1).

Table 4.1 Effect of injury on resting metabolic expenditure

Healthy individual at rest	25 kcal/kg
Healthy individual + walking	+20%
Uncomplicated surgery, e.g. vagotomy	+10%
Multiple fractures	+10–20%
Major surgery + sepsis, e.g. peritonitis	+25–50%
Major burns	+50–100%

Figures quoted as % healthy individual at rest.

Glucose metabolism

Tissues undergoing repair appear to use glucose preferentially as respiratory substrate and the raised concentrations of catabolic hormones associated with the stress situation (glucagon, catecholamines and cortisol) may be a result of an adaptive response to answer the requirement for glucose by stimulating gluconeogenesis (Fig. 4.2). In general the increase in blood glucose reflects the severity of injury. However, the high rate of metabolism is generally a wasteful process delaying recovery.

The secretion of insulin by the pancreatic β-cells returns to normal in the flow phase and insulin levels may even be raised above normal although not as high as would be expected for the given glucose load. Peripheral insulin

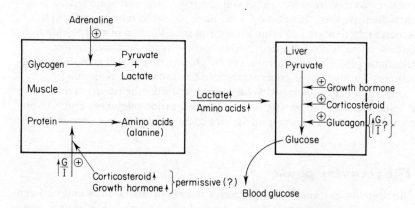

Fig. 4.2 Hormonal and metabolic changes during the flow phase.

resistance is still evident at this time, again as a result of cortisol antagonism and raised plasma free fatty acid concentrations, so that glucose entry into peripheral tissues is reduced. A glucose tolerance test at this stage is also abnormal and resembles that of the maturity onset diabetic, i.e. lowered tolerance and a reduced glucose lowering effect of insulin.

Protein metabolism

Of particular importance during the flow phase is the loss of lean body mass. Despite a pronounced hyperglycaemia, gluconeogenesis from muscle amino acids is increased and patients show a negative nitrogen balance. The lack of the protein sparing effect of insulin and the catabolic action of cortisol on muscle protein result in increased muscle protein breakdown providing substrate for anabolic processes stimulated by glucagon and cortisol in liver. This increased breakdown of muscle protein is responsible for the increased nitrogen excretion seen in the flow phase. The muscle itself appears to catabolize preferentially branched chain amino acids, transaminating the nitrogen to pyruvate derived from glucose or to glutamate. Alanine then serves as a carrier to the liver of waste nitrogen and 3 carbon units for gluconeogenesis.

Fat metabolism

Although protein breakdown is increased to provide substrate for gluconeogenesis, it does not become the major source of calories even after severe injury. Studies on resting energy expenditure and nitrogen balance in patients who had undergone a variety of surgical operations suggested that even in cases where nitrogen excretion was greatly increased, e.g. massive soft tissue injury, protein contributed only 20–25 per cent of total calories. Under these extreme catabolic conditions, as in starvation, body fat was still the major endogenous energy source. The increase in serum free fatty acid concentration is proportional to the severity of the injury and many tissues continue to use free fatty acid as respiratory substrate despite a high carbohydrate load. Intralipid for instance is cleared more rapidly in the hypercatabolic state following injury and mobilization of triglyceride from adipose tissue is not inhibited by the existing hyperglycaemia, raised circulating insulin concentration or by glucose intake as it is in the fasting patient. This increased concentration of free fatty acids available for oxidation leads to increased ketogenesis but unlike the situation in starvation is insufficient to compensate for the non-utilization of glucose and is unable to prevent continued muscle protein breakdown and gluconeogenesis.

The recovery phase

Nitrogen loss as a result of depletion of muscle protein is maximal between 4 to 8 days after simple injury such as long bone fracture and is usually less than 60–70 g. In more severe cases which may involve secondary infections, for example major burns, the total nitrogen loss may exceed 300 g and of course loss of such an enormous amount of lean body mass may be critical. Besides providing substrates for gluconeogenesis, amino acids derived from muscle protein breakdown may also be used in the hepatic synthesis of plasma proteins whose concentrations rise after injury, the acute phase reactants such as C-reactive protein, acid α_1-glycoprotein, α_1-antitrypsin and fibrinogen. Amino acids will also be required in the flow phase for the synthesis of those proteins whose concentration falls after trauma. For example, serum albumin concentration may fall by as much as 30 per cent after severe surgery, probably due to changes in the permeability of the capillary membrane leading to leakage of albumin from the intravascular into the interstitial space. Synthesis of such proteins both acute phase reactants and other plasma proteins occurs even when exogenous nutritional support for the patient is often difficult.

As stated earlier the return to homoeostasis may be a prolonged process as the body gradually adjusts to the demand of the metabolic changes brought about by the injury. An understanding of these metabolic changes has enabled improved management of the patient during the shock and hypermetabolic phases particularly through the nutritional support to the patient. Diets tailor-made for a specific patient may be prepared and thus problems of over- or underfeeding and of perhaps misfeeding may be obviated. Such specific nutritional support is critical for recovery during the flow phase and for replacement of lean body mass in the final anabolic stage.

Although the present account is not meant to be an over-simplification of the metabolic events following injury, in many cases the situation may be further complicated by sepsis and the previous nutritional status of the patient. An increased resting energy expenditure is associated with major infections and this is in addition to that produced by the injury itself. Poorly nourished patients have little labile protein available for catabolism in the flow phase and thus may be unable to survive even a modest weight loss as a result of major trauma.

5

Exercise

During exercise the chemical energy of ATP is converted by muscle into mechanical energy (work). Ultimately all our chemical energy is derived from the oxidation of food-stuffs and body stores using the process of oxidative phosphorylation and thus all exercise is accompanied by increased body O_2 consumption. This can rise 10- to 20-fold in the change from resting to intense exercise. The increased metabolic activity implied by this rise in O_2 intake is not exclusively confined to the muscles involved in exercise since both heart action and ventilation rate increase considerably and the metabolic co-operation of other tissues such as adipose and liver are required for the maintenance or replenishment of muscle fuel stores. Muscle, unlike any other tissue, is called upon to support massive increases in metabolic flux (up to 1000-fold), often in extremely short periods. The control of metabolism in muscle is therefore tightly geared to the maintenance and provision of sufficient ATP for muscle contraction. This chapter will discuss the control of skeletal muscle metabolism and its links with metabolic control in the other tissues in the two situations of first maximal effort that can be maintained for short periods of around 2 to 3 minutes (anaerobic exercise) and second exercise that can be maintained for much longer periods (aerobic exercise).

The terms anaerobic and aerobic relate to the metabolic processes which generate the ATP actually used by the working muscle. Anaerobic processes comprise the reactions 1. and 2. below:

1. Creatine phosphate + ADP → creatine + ATP
2. Glycogen + ADP + P_i → lactate + ATP

Aerobic processes are those involving oxidative phosphorylation:

$$2H \text{ (from various substrates)} + O + 3ADP + 3P_i \rightarrow 3ATP + H_2O$$

In aerobic and anaerobic exercise different muscle fibre types are recruited. Human skeletal muscle consists of a mixture of fibre types but they can be broadly classified into two groups (Table 5.1) differing in capacity for energy generation (measured by enzyme content), lipid stores and contractile properties. Type I, with slower contraction time, higher oxidative capacity, greater lipid stores and capillary supply is used in prolonged aerobic exercise whereas type II with faster contraction time and high glycolytic capacity is

Table 5.1   Human muscle fibre types

Property	Type I (red)	Type II (white)
Myoglobin content	+ +	+/−
Anaerobic energy generation	+	+ +
Aerobic energy generation	+ +	+/−
Myofibrillar ATPase	+	+ +
Contraction time	+	+ +
Glycogen content	+ +	+ +
Triglyceride content	+ +	+/−
Major recruitment	Prolonged exercise	Intense exercise
Capillary supply	+ +	+

mainly involved in anaerobic exercise. However in both muscle fibre types
the activities of oxidative and glycolytic enzymes are large enough to allow
significant aerobic and anaerobic metabolism to proceed.

Anaerobic exercise

Initial stimulus of glycolysis

In the resting skeletal muscle the energy needs of the tissue are filled by the
oxidation of blood-borne substrates, primarily fatty acids, ketone bodies and
glucose. But during the first few seconds of light to moderate exercise and for
all of short-duration heavy exercise, ATP is produced anaerobically from
muscle stores of creatine phosphate and glycogen. This occurs because the
demand for ATP exceeds the ability of oxidative phosphorylation to supply
it. At the onset of exercise the rate of use of ATP may increase by 100- to
1000-fold and the extra O_2 needed by the muscle to generate this ATP by
oxidative phosphorylation is not present. Even in red muscle the
oxymyoglobin content is not sufficient to regenerate more than one-fifth of
the resting muscle ATP content (Table 5.2). Thus ATP is initially

Table 5.2   Skeletal muscle energy reserves

Compound	Content (μmol/g wet weight)	Max. ATP equivalent (μmol/g wet weight)
ATP	5	5
Creatine phosphate	30	30
Myoglobin	0.2	1
Glycogen glucose	80–100	2000 (anaerobic)
		38 000 (aerobic)
Triglyceride	5–15	412 000

replenished at the expense of creatine phosphate. As this proceeds critical
changes take place in the ratios of concentrations of activator and inhibitor
molecules of the phosphofructokinase reaction. In the resting state the
concentrations of inhibitors of this enzyme (ATP, creatine phosphate and
citrate) are high in relation to the activators (AMP, NH_4^+ and fructose-

1,6 bisphosphate). During initiation of muscle activity the concentration of inhibitors fall while that of activators rise. In particular a small decrease in the ATP/ADP ratio causes a much larger increase in concentration of AMP and NH_4^+ via the following extremely active process:

$$2ADP \rightleftharpoons ATP + AMP$$
$$AMP + H_2O \rightarrow IMP + NH_4^+$$

Thus AMP and NH_4^+ concentrations increase in proportion to the square of the ADP concentration. This allows rapid activation of phosphofructokinase and greatly stimulates glycolysis resulting in lactate accumulation and regeneration of ATP from ADP.

Initiation of glycogen breakdown

The main glycolytic fuel during initiation of exercise or during high intensity heavy exercise is muscle glycogen. The signal for breakdown of glycogen stores is two-fold: first an increase in the ratio of concentration of allosteric activator (AMP) to inhibitors (ATP, glucose-6-phosphate) of phosphorylase **b** and second increased concentrations of cyclic AMP (cAMP) and Ca^{2+} in the muscle resulting from elevation of plasma catecholamines and from nervous stimulation of the muscle fibres respectively. The former signal allows activation of the dephosphorylated **b** form of phosphorylase by 'energy related' metabolites. In resting muscle this enzyme is largely inactive due to the low ratio of AMP to ATP and glucose-6-phosphate but as explained in the previous section the onset of muscle activity increases the content of AMP resulting in stimulation of glycogen breakdown. The increased concentrations of cAMP and Ca^{2+} both result in activation of phosphorylase **b** kinase and the conversion of phosphorylase **b** to **a** allowing rapid glycogen breakdown independently of any energy related feedback. Thus the signal for muscle contraction is co-ordinated with that for glycogen breakdown allowing mobilization of the fuel necessary to maintain the exercise. Raised catecholamines play a necessary part in sudden 'fight or flight' responses but are less important in the early phase of anticipated exercise. Fig. 5.1 summarizes the co-ordination of muscle contraction with glycogen mobilization and glycolysis. This sequence of events applies to all muscle types when exercise is initiated; what happens after the initial period depends largely on the intensity of exercise and the resulting ATP demand.

The onset of exercise is associated with increased heart rate, in part at least due to nerve reflexes routed from the exercising skeletal muscle to the cardiac regulation centre of the brain. Increase in heart action allows greater blood flow to the working muscle. This can rise 100-fold during the first minute of exercise and thus the rate of delivery of O_2 to the muscle and subsequent oxidative phosphorylation can increase markedly. But in intensely exercising muscle the requirement for ATP per unit time exceeds the rate at which O_2 and blood borne substrates are delivered and results in the maintenance of high rates of glycolysis at the expense of muscle glycogen (Fig. 5.1). Glycogen breakdown is increased at high work rates since release of catecholamines is stimulated. This allows a continued high rate of ATP supply by glycolysis.

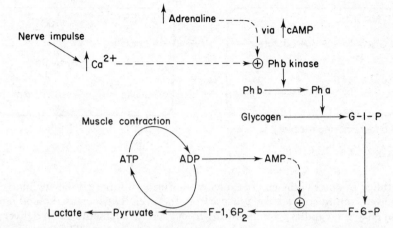

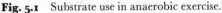

Fig. 5.1 Substrate use in anaerobic exercise.

Limits to anaerobic exercise

High intensity anaerobic exercise can only continue for a limited period. Ultimately muscle glycogen content (Table 5.2) supports maximal glycolysis for not more than 3 to 4 minutes. More commonly the limit is imposed by the accumulation of lactate. During intense exercise this is formed at a very rapid rate, faster than the rate of removal by the capillary network even allowing for increased blood flow. The result is a drop in muscle pH to around 6.6. At this pH, phosphofructokinase is more sensitive to inhibition by its allosteric effectors thus resulting in reduced glycolytic rate and decreased work capacity. In addition H^+ competes with Ca^{2+} for binding to troponin (a protein required for the Ca^{2+} stimulation of muscle contraction) thus decreasing muscle force.

Oxygen debt and regeneration of substrate stores

During any exercise there is an increase in heart rate, blood flow and ventilation with increased O_2 consumption. However during 'anaerobic' exercise the major part of the increased O_2 consumption occurs after the exercise has ended. Here an O_2 'debt' is incurred by the use of anaerobic mechanisms for the generation of ATP during the period of exercise. As soon as exercise ceases the continuing increased flow of blood-borne O_2 is now sufficient to allow rephosphorylation of ADP by oxidative processes so that part of the extra O_2 consumption will be due to topping up supplies of ATP and creatine phosphate with resultant inhibition of glycolysis.

The major part of the O_2 debt is involved in replenishing muscle glycogen via hepatic gluconeogenesis as part of the operation of the Cori cycle (Fig. 5.2). Both liver and muscle glycogen stores will suffer depletion during anaerobic exercise since catecholamine release is stimulated and this activates phosphorylase in liver allowing increased release of hepatic glycogen as glucose. The elevated plasma levels of catecholamines return to normal

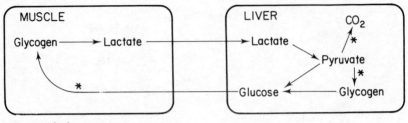

* occurs during recovery

Fig. 5.2 The Cori cycle.

within 6 minutes of the end of exercise but during this period they will have allowed continued release of glucose from the liver. The increased blood flow and enlarged capillary area resulting from exercise augment insulin delivery to muscle allowing glucose entry and glycogen reformation. The lactate released from muscle is in part oxidized by liver while the rest is used to fill the liver glycogen deficit.

Diet and muscle glycogen content

The muscle glycogen content depends to some extent on the diet. Intense exercise periods on a low carbohydrate diet will deplete the glycogen in the exercising muscles but subsequent refeeding on high carbohydrate allows an overshoot to occur in which glycogen levels can reach up to 3 times normal values in those muscles which had been exercised. This has formed the basis for dietary procedures designed to improve performance in athletic events.

Aerobic exercise

Oxygen availability and $\dot{V}_{O_2 max}$

Aerobic exercise occurs at lower work intensities than those requiring anaerobic ATP regeneration and is the characteristic mode for exercise carried out over longer periods. After the initial burst of anaerobic ATP regeneration associated with the onset of any bout of exercise, the increased O_2 supply to the working muscle can support a substantial increase in cell respiration and ATP synthesis by oxidative phosphorylation. Because of the greater efficiency of this mode of ATP production this level of work can be sustained for very considerable periods.

The maximum of intensity of work supported by aerobic ATP production must however be limited by tissue oxygenation. In effect therefore the principal limitation for exercise lasting more than 4 minutes is the capacity of the heart and circulation to deliver O_2 to the working muscles. In any individual the rate of maximal oxygen uptake ($\dot{V}_{O_2 max}$) is a measure of this limit. Expressed as ml of O_2/min/kg of body weight $\dot{V}_{O_2 max}$ would be around 40 to 50 for female and male medical students respectively. Since aerobic exercise is limited by oxygen delivery rate it follows that any rate of working which exceeds that requiring the $\dot{V}_{O_2max}$ will involve some anaerobic energy generation and will therefore increase the rate at which muscle glycogen deposits are depleted and reduce endurance. Thus competitive track events run over distances up to 3000 metres involve some anaerobic contribution the greatest being found in those (100 and 200 metres) run at the highest speed. Events such as the 10 000 metres and marathon (42.2 km) are exclusively aerobic in character.

Available fuels and their relative merits

Although muscle contains only limited amounts of fuel (Table 5.2) the longer time scale of aerobic exercise allows hormonal and metabolic changes to occur which give access to blood-borne glucose (from hepatic glycogen or gluconeogenic precursors) and fatty acids and ketone bodies (derived ultimately from adipose tissue triglyceride). However an important difference should be noted in the oxidative use of glucose and fatty acids. Since the limitation on the rate of work is the rate of oxygen supply it follows that high power aerobic exercise (approaching $\dot{V}_{O_2max}$) is best supported by the substrate requiring the lease number of molecules of O_2 per molecule of ATP generated.

Compare the oxidation of glucose and a fatty acid:

$$glucose + 6O_2 \rightarrow 6CO_2 + H_2O + 38\ ATP$$
$$palmitic\ acid\ (C_{16}) + 23O_2 \rightarrow 16CO_2 + 16H_2O + 130\ ATP$$

For highest power generation carbohydrate derived fuel is about 12 per cent better than fat derived fuel in terms of O_2 required per ATP. It is thus found that aerobic exercise at high power (>90 per cent of $\dot{V}_{O_2max}$) is associated with maximum use and depletion of muscle glycogen. However, when one considers ATP yields per molecule or ATP generated per unit weight of fuel, oxidation of carbohydrate is 30 per cent to 50 per cent less efficient respectively than fatty acid. For maximal aerobic endurance fat is therefore the most efficient source of fuel and in events such as the marathon a considerable use of fatty acid has been demonstrated. However it must be stressed that no fuel is used exclusively in aerobic metabolism. Muscle consumes all fuels available, the only differences being in the time scale and the relative rates of their consumption.

Hormonal changes

The mobilization and use of these fuels is controlled by the hormonal changes occurring during exercise (Table 5.3).

Adrenaline and noradrenaline (catecholamines) produced by the adrenal medulla and sympathetic nervous system respectively are found to rise in concentration in plasma as soon as the work intensity is sufficient to require an O_2 uptake of around 60 per cent of $\dot{V}_{O_2max}$. The increase continues with rising work intensity through the aerobic/anaerobic threshold at 100 per cent $\dot{V}_{O2max}$. Noradrenaline concentration is usually higher than adrenaline in

Table 5.3   Hormonal changes with exercise

Hormone	Plasma change	Type of exercise
Catecholamine	↑	Intense (anaerobic or aerobic)
Insulin	↓	Intense, prolonged aerobic
Glucagon	↑	Prolonged aerobic
Growth hormone	↑	Prolonged aerobic

exercise indicating the important contribution of the sympathetic nervous system. Apart from stimulation of cardiac output, these two hormones exert a major effect on the mobilization of muscle glycogen as well as stimulating adipose tissue lipolysis and contributing to the stimulation of liver glycogenolysis.

Plasma insulin concentrations fall during exercise and the magnitude of the change (as with catecholamines) depends on the intensity and duration of the exercise. This may reflect a role of the sympathetic nervous system inhibiting insulin secretion via α-adrenergic receptors on the β-cells. Decreased insulin concentration plays a role in reducing all those anaerobic processes (glycogen synthesis, fatty acid synthesis, triglyceride synthesis) that would compete or interfere with substrate mobilization.

The other hormones whose concentrations change significantly in aerobic exercise are glucagon, glucocorticoids (cortisol) and growth hormone. Their concentrations increase only after prolonged submaximal exercise or shorter periods of heavy aerobic work. The effects of glucagon are primarily to stimulate hepatic gluconeogenesis and glycogenolysis while cortisol and growth hormone increase adipose tissue lipolysis with cortisol stimulating gluconeogenesis in liver as well.

In summary these responses serve to mobilize muscle and body fuel reserves of glycogen and fat and to stimulate necessary processes such as hepatic gluconeogenesis and uptake of gluconeogenic precursors.

Substrate utilization in aerobic exercise (Fig. 5.3)

Under the conditions of prolonged activity at submaximal rates of work (50–70 per cent of $\dot{V}_{O_2max}$, e.g. marathon running) the substrates consumed by working muscles are: muscle glycogen and triglyceride, blood-borne fatty acid and ketone bodies and blood-borne glucose. Initially, under the influence of raised concentrations of catecholamines, oxidation of glucose predominates, the glucose deriving in part from muscle glycogen and in part from liver glycogen. However, oxidation of fatty acids (which provide a significant part of resting muscle's fuel) is stimulated by the increase in lipolysis caused by the raised catecholamines. The significant rate of fatty acid and ketone body oxidation in muscle has a sparing effect on glucose oxidation (raised citrate inhibiting glycolysis at phosphofructokinase and raised acetyl-CoA and NADH inhibiting pyruvate dehydrogenase). Biopsy of exercising human muscle has shown that the major part of muscle glycogen consumption occurs in the first 60 minutes of prolonged exercise. The decrease in this period is around 50 per cent of the glycogen initially present.

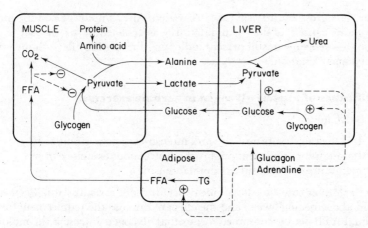

Fig. 5.3 Substrate use in prolonged (aerobic) exercise.

In the first 60 minutes the concentration of insulin has dropped significantly reinforcing the catabolic effect of the raised catecholamines on lipolysis and hepatic glycogenolysis. But in spite of this drop in insulin concentration, muscle uptake of glucose actually increases so that oxidation of blood-borne glucose can contribute up to 37 per cent of O_2 consumption at this time. The increased uptake of glucose by muscle is due to two effects:

1. An augmented rate of insulin delivery to exercising muscle due to the greatly increased blood flow.
2. An absolute increase in the transport of glucose into exercising muscle independent of insulin concentration.

In this context it has been known for many years that physical exertion increased glucose uptake and utilization in muscle of insulin-withdrawn diabetics.

Glucose metabolism by exercising muscle lowers arterial glucose concentrations and this coincides with the rise in plasma glucagon, cortisol and growth hormone which becomes significant after about 1 hour of exercise. The consequences of these changes are further glycogenolysis in liver and 2-fold increased hepatic gluconeogenesis. Substrates for gluconeogenesis are lactate and alanine both of which are derived from accumulating pyruvate in muscle whose oxidation is spared by increased acetyl-CoA provision from fatty acid and ketone body oxidation. The raised glucagon level stimulates hepatic extraction of alanine causing a drop in the concentration of the latter in arterial blood during prolonged exercise. The amino group of alanine is derived from transamination in muscle cells of branched-chain amino acids derived from liver and muscle protein.

As the period of exercise continues beyond 2 hours the metabolism of glucose by the working muscle decreases due to the considerable fatty acid oxidation now occurring in this tissue. Glucose is thus spared for oxidation by brain. The extent of fat oxidation by submaximally working muscle has been shown by analysis of biopsy samples taken from participants in the arduous

86 km Vasa cross-country ski race in Sweden. After 7 hours of exercise the triglyceride content of the vastus lateralis was depleted by 50 per cent although glycogen was still present indicating the sparing effect on the latter of fatty acid oxidation.

Significance of muscle glycogen in aerobic exercise

This is two fold:

1. It is the major substrate at work intensities $>$ 90 per cent of $\dot{V}_{O_2max}$
2. It determines the duration for which strenuous exercise can be maintained even at submaximal intensities.

In the former case catecholamine concentrations are substantially elevated (4-fold above resting levels) and the effect of this and the requirement for maximal ATP per O_2 consumed means that glycogen glucose is the major fuel oxidized. At 90 per cent of $\dot{V}_{O_2max}$ the muscle glycogen stores would be depleted in about 60 minutes. The mechanism of the switch to glycogen in the presence of more than adequate supplies of fatty acid is not clear but may be connected with increased recruitment of type II fibres at work rates 90 per cent $\dot{V}_{O_2max}$. In these fibres an increased demand for ATP would be met by increased provision of pyruvate from glycogen since they have less fatty acid oxidative ability than type I fibres (see Table 5.1). When muscle glycogen stores are depleted the exercise must either stop or it must be reduced in intensity. This phenomenon is known amongst marathon runners as 'hitting the wall'.

Effects of training

Endurance training causes increased protein synthesis in heart muscle and the muscles undergoing exercise. In heart muscle this results in hypertrophy and increased maximal cardial output (due to a greater stroke volume) but no increase in heart rate. There is also no change in the oxidative capacity of heart tissue. In skeletal muscle however there is a 2–3 fold rise in mitochondrial content and metabolic capacity especially towards oxidation of fatty acids and ketone bodies. Additionally the myoglobin content of muscle is increased thus aiding O_2 entry, storage and transport to mitochondria. Taken together, these effects account for the more than 2-fold increase in $\dot{V}_{O_2max}$ seen on training.

It is however noteworthy that muscle glycogen does not increase in training and neither does the activity of the enzymes involved in breakdown of glycogen to pyruvate. But liver glycogen doubles in amount as does the activity of muscle hexokinase indicating an important role for blood-borne glucose in sparing the glycogen of exercising muscle. Similarly the adaptive increase in capacity to oxidize fatty acids and ketone bodies results in inhibition of glycogen metabolism and greater reliance on fat reserves when trained. In addition this adaptation decreases the production of lactate resulting in a slower rate of tiring. The accumulation of lactate is also reduced as a result of the greater capillarization of muscle on training allowing an increased perfusion of the tissue and transport of the lactate to the liver by the circulation.

The trained individual can thus exercise at higher absolute work rates for longer periods than the untrained. At submaximal intensities he can make more efficient use of all the fuels available causing a smaller disturbance to glucose homoeostasis and slower use of muscle glycogen. This results in greater endurance during exercise and a more rapid recovery after exercise in the case of the trained athlete.

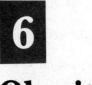

Obesity

The maintenance of a relatively stable body weight, such as is seen in the majority of individuals, requires some element of homoeostatic control where caloric intake is exactly balanced by caloric expenditure. An excess of as little as 1 per cent in intake over expenditure would result in a body weight gain in excess of 1000 kg after an allotted life span of three score years and ten! A number of observations have suggested that body weight and composition are maintained physiologically at a predetermined 'set point' in a manner analogous to other body parameters e.g. temperature. For instance, as many would-be slimmers will verify, maintenance of a new, decreased body weight is extremely difficult. On the other hand, young rats whose weight had been manipulated by artificial feeding regimes re-established ideal weight for age once returned to normal feeding habits. Similarly medical students fed 2000 kcal each night for one month via a nasogastric tube showed no alteration in their daily food intake and surprisingly did not gain weight. Such observations imply that body weight is a strictly regulated parameter and within certain limits differences in caloric intake or expenditure can be accommodated. A close relationship between the regulation of intake and expenditure must exist (Table 6.1.).

Table 6.1 Possible regulators of a stable body weight

Energy intake	Energy output
1. Psychological factors	1. Metabolic energy expenditure
2. Social factors	2. Dietary induced thermogenesis
3. Physiological factors	3. Mechanical energy expenditure
(a) gastric distension	
(b) neurological centres of feeding control	
4. Biochemical factors	
(a) Gastrointestinal hormones	
(b) steroid hormone ratio	

Control of caloric intake

The mechanisms controlling eating are poorly understood. Food intake is probably influenced by the combined interaction of a variety of factors, physiological, biochemical and psycho-social. Studies of responses after CNS ablation suggest that feeding and satiety centres exist in the hypothalamic region. It is also probable that the limbic system and more specifically the amygdaloid body are involved in feeding control since destruction of this area in monkeys is associated with the Kluver–Bucy syndrome characterized by insatiable appetite and increased aggressive sexual behaviour. Mechanical gastric distension, with the accompanying feeling of fulness, may also be an important feature of satiety.

Nutritional receptors in the GI tract for substances such as dietary lipids, proteins and carbohydrates are known to control the luminal secretion of digestive enzymes such as proteases, lipases and amylases. These receptors also control the release of a range of gastro-intestinal peptide hormones which may affect the systemic release of endocrine agents such as insulin and glucagon, and thus modify the 'direction' of the body's metabolism. In addition many of these gastro-intestinal hormones act as powerful peripheral and central neuromodulatory agents (e.g. substance P, vasoactive intestinal polypeptide, somatostatin and neurotensin). Such actions have led to speculation that some or all of these hormones play a role in the modulation of feeding habits. It is possible that a GI-CNS axis exists by which the drive for nutritional elements is influenced by the release of hormones from the GI tract in response to the presence of food in the lumen.

Steroid hormones have also been suggested as regulators of body weight, composition, and fat distribution. The conversion of androgenic steroids to oestrogens occurs in adipose tissue and an increase in adipose tissue mass might be expected to increase the ratio of oestrogens to androgens. Such change in hormonal levels might be important in modulating feeding behaviour and caloric expenditure. (See Table 6.1.)

Psychological and social influences may also have major effects on eating behaviour in man. Caloric intake is affected significantly by social environment (e.g. frequency of dinner parties), cultural norms (e.g. third world versus first world) and psychological state (e.g. eating for solace or from boredom). Visual 'clues' appear to be important in determining just how much food is to be consumed since we often feel 'full' when we have eaten what appears visually to be an adequate amount of food.

Control of caloric expenditure

Caloric expenditure may be divided into two main categories—metabolic expenditure and mechanical expenditure.

Metabolic expenditure

Metabolic output, formally called basal metabolic rate, is a parameter dependent on a wide range of variable factors which include:

1. The ratio of body size to surface area; smaller individuals have higher metabolic rates.

2. Age; at birth the metabolic rate is low, rises to a maximum at about 5 years of age and subsequently decreases with age.

3. Sex; women have slower metabolic rates than men.

4. Metabolic status as related to health; metabolic rate increases in disease.

5. Nutritional intake; as calorie intake decreases so also does metabolic activity and thus starvation does not necessarily produce the expected rapid weight loss (i.e. a decreased caloric intake is compensated for by a fall in metabolic caloric expenditure). The relationship between caloric intake and expenditure by metabolism was first described by Rubner who showed that dogs fed with food of a known caloric value expended a quantifiable amount of calories as heat. This was referred to as the 'specific dynamic action'. Low caloric intake resulted in heat production which exceeded the caloric value of the ingested foods and gives credence to the slimmer's slogan 'eat little and often rather than all in one go'. Such an effect is also responsible for the feeling of warmth after eating a meal (postprandial hyperthermia). This phenomenon has become known as dietary induced thermogenesis (DIT) and may involve one or all of the following:

(a) *Release of noradrenaline.* The presence of food in the GI tract causes certain cells to release noradrenaline into the systemic portal circulation. This catabolic hormone stimulates glycogen and triglyceride breakdown and their subsequent oxidation. Such an inappropriate use of metabolic fuel is wasteful and increases caloric expenditure. Noradrenaline also directly stimulates fat catabolism in brown adipose tissue.

(b) *Futile cycling.* This is the term given to the non-productive flux of substrates through a series of anabolic and catabolic reactions with the consequential dissipation of energy as heat. Possible futile cycles are listed in Fig. 6.1. Such cycles are thought to be particularly important in insects such as bees, where the 'primary' heating of flight muscle is essential for the efficient functioning of the muscle. Although theoretically possible in man the role of futile cycles in DIT remains uncertain.

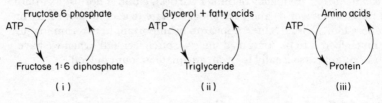

(i)   (ii)   (iii)

Fig. 6.1   Possible futile cycles.

(c) *Brown adipose tissue metabolism.* The oxidation of substrates in the mitochondrion produces NADH and $FADH_2$ (in the citric acid cycle and β-oxidation). Oxidation of these coenzymes in turn by the electron transport chain on the inner mitochondrial membrane creates a transmitochondrial proton gradient (across the inner membrane). Re-entry of protons into the matrix via a specific membrane carrier utilizes the potential energy of this

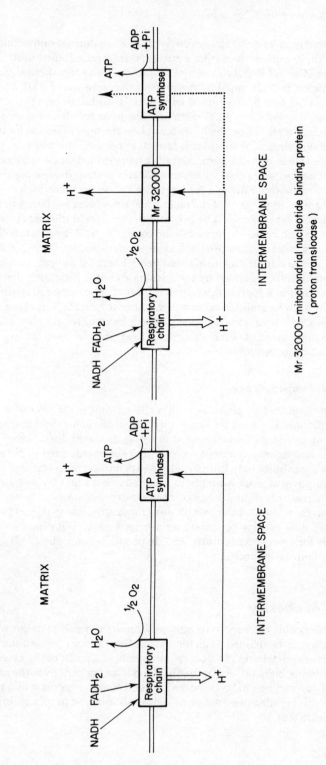

Fig. 6.2 Links between respiration and ATP synthesis in (a) normal and (b) brown adipose tissue mitochondria.

(a) NORMAL MITOCHONDRIA

(b) BROWN ADIPOSE TISSUE MITOCHONDRIA

MATRIX

INTERMEMBRANE SPACE

NADH FADH₂

H₂O

½ O₂

Respiratory
chain

H⁺

H⁺

ADP
+Pi

ATP

ATP
synthase

Mr 32000 – mitochondrial nucleotide binding protein
(proton translocase)

proton motive force to drive the synthesis of ATP. In normal mitochondria (Fig. 6.2a) the energy derived from nutritional substrates is used quite efficiently to form ATP and this acts to inhibit oxidative metabolism (i.e. the rate of oxidation is determined by the matrix concentration of ADP). Such mitochondria are said to be coupled with NADH oxidation being stoichiometrically linked to ATP synthesis. The mitochondria of brown adipose tissue (Fig. 6.2b) on the other hand become uncoupled under the influence of noradrenaline stimulated fatty acid release. The inner membranes of these mitochondria contain a specific nucleotide binding protein (subunit m.w. 32 000) which translocates protons dissipating the proton gradient without driving ATP synthesis. This protein which constitutes about 10 per cent of the membrane proteins is not found in the mitochondria of other tissues. The presence of the protein thus short circuits ATP synthesis and removes the metabolic control of oxidative metabolism. Oxidation of substrates then proceeds at an accelerated, uncontrolled rate, the energy released from such oxidations being liberated as heat. Catabolic processes are usually regulated by the adenylate charge ratio such that when ATP concentration is high catabolism is inhibited. The failure to synthesize ATP despite a high catabolic rate ensures continued catabolism. Thus lipid catabolic flux in brown adipose tissue proceeds in an unregulated manner such that a large amount of metabolic fuel (food) may be oxidized to produce heat without contributing to body mass.

Mechanical expenditure

Utilization of calories by physical work is also a factor in the overall energy balance equation. For instance heavy physical work such as felling trees might use up to 12 kcal/min compared to 1 kcal/min used during sleep. However it has become apparent recently that the energy used in physical work *per se* contributes only little to caloric expenditure. It is probable that the effect of physical work is simply to raise the individual's level of fitness and thus increase his resting metabolic caloric expenditure.

Although each of the above mechanisms might contribute to energy expenditure their relative contributions are not known. With these possibilities for energy expenditure why do people become obese? Can a regulatory fault be identified?

Causes of obesity

While obese people are easy to recognize it is more difficult to define obesity. Generally it may be defined as an increase in body weight beyond the limitations of skeletal and physical requirements as a result of the excessive accumulation of body fat. An individual who is 20 per cent over the ideal weight for age and height is considered obese. Obesity may arise as a result of rare congenital syndromes, endocrinological disorders or simply chronic over-eating (Table 6.2).

Table 6.2 Potential causes of obesity

1. Rare congenital syndromes with associated obesity

2. Changes in endocrinological status
   (a) Anabolic hormones
   (b) Catabolic hormones

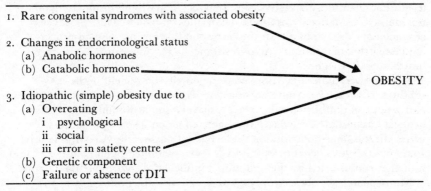

OBESITY

3. Idiopathic (simple) obesity due to
   (a) Overeating
       i   psychological
       ii social
       iii error in satiety centre
   (b) Genetic component
   (c) Failure or absence of DIT

Rare congenital syndromes

Obesity occurs as one of the symptoms of conditions such as Frohlich's syndrome, Stein–Leventhal syndrome and the Laurence–Moon–Beidl syndrome. Despite their attractive names these conditions are extremely rare and a discussion of them is beyond the scope of the present text.

Endocrinological disorders

Disruptions of hormonal balance which promote the action of anabolic hormones, inhibit the action of catabolic hormones or both will lead to increased body weight. Thus high concentrations of insulin (hyperinsulinaemia) promote fatty acid and triglyceride synthesis in adipose tissue and glycogen synthesis in liver and muscle (Table 9.2). Similarly disruption of pituitary function leading to increased growth hormone or prolactin secretion can induce an anabolic state. Alterations in steroid hormone levels as found in Cushing's syndrome, pregnancy and gonadal dysfunction may also stimulate fat deposition. In contrast, a reduction in the concentration of catabolic hormones may have a similar effect, e.g. hypothyroidism in adults is associated with obesity. Such endocrine disorders are amenable to therapy and the obesity regresses with appropriate treatment. However as with the congenital syndromes obesity due to readily identifiable endocrine disorders is rather uncommon.

Simple obesity

Most people who are obese fall into the category of simple obesity. The category is a misnomer since it describes a very complex state which is not well understood. Measurement of circulating hormone concentrations in obese subjects occasionally indicates a disturbance of the endocrine balance such as has been mentioned above but such hormonal disturbances are usually a result of rather than the cause of, the obesity. Weight reduction by dietary or other means, invariably leads to a return to normal hormone levels. For example, in obesity-associated secondary hyperinsulinaemia there is a marked resistance to insulin in the peripheral tissues. This resistance is a characteristic of the obese state and is responsible for the compensatory hypersecretion of insulin. A loss of resistance to insulin occurs on return to 'normal' body weight.

Sibling twin studies have implicated a genetic component in the production of the obese state but the hereditary pattern is extremely complex and is not compatible with the conveyance of a single dominant or recessive gene. It has been described as a multigene function whereby a number of genes effect a small contribution to the overall obese state. A comprehensive study of the role of genetics in obesity is severely limited by its complexity and is further complicated by the undoubted influence of environmental factors.

Many people are obese simply because of over-eating especially as a consequence of social and environmental pressures to which the individual may be subjected, e.g. chefs being surrounded by food; businessmen taking working lunches. It may also be a consequence of socially accepted norms where 'fat is beautiful', or due to emotional or psychological problems which cause aberrant eating behaviour, e.g. pre-examination nerves. There may however be a more fundamental fault in the perception of satiety in the obese individual. For instance obese people draw more of a fluid meal and are significantly less satisfied than their lean counterparts when fed from a hidden reservoir of liquid food. Similarly obese people appear incapable of adjusting intake to compensate for changes in the caloric value of food. This loss of control of intake is possibly due to a malfunction in the CNS.

More recently it has been suggested that many people become obese because of a decreased ability to convert metabolic fuels to heat. Their capacity for dietary-induced thermogenesis appears markedly decreased in comparison to lean controls, carbohydrate, fat and protein being stored as glycogen or fat rather than oxidized wastefully. Obese individuals appear to have significantly less brown adipose tissue (the site of DIT) than lean individuals and as such may well be victims of their own metabolic efficiency.

Clinical aspects of obesity

Obesity is essentially a problem of the overfed civilized world, being relatively uncommon in third world countries. Using the strict definition of obesity, on p. 52, up to 40 per cent of the population of the USA could be considered obese. The condition carries a significant increase in mortality and disorders such as diabetes mellitus, respiratory insufficiency (Pickwickian syndrome), hypertension, atheroma and thromboembolic disease are complications of obesity which carry significant mortality risks. In addition the quality of life of an obese individual may be reduced by such problems as gallstones, osteoarthritis, skeletal strain, varicose veins, hernias and possible depression. Obesity should not be overlooked as a precipitating factor of illness.

Treatment of the obese patient

Treatments of obesity are relatively ineffective probably because of the often multifactorial nature of the problem.

Reduction of caloric intake

Dieting is an obvious treatment in the short term but, unless psychological and social problems are also addressed, may not be successful in the long term. Some help may be gained from 'slimming with others' as a member of a weight-watching group. But even so a clear understanding of the problem and the implications of being chronically overweight should be given. Although initial weight reduction is rapid and quite marked due to the mobilization of part of the glycogen store and its associated water, further weight loss is a slow process. Glycogen has a caloric value of 4 kcal/g and is stored in muscle and liver with water in a ratio of 1:3 (glycogen:water). Thus utilization of 1 g of glycogen (4 kcal) results in a 4 g decrease in body weight. However in the obese individual excess weight is stored as triglyceride and in order to reduce weight significantly this must be burned off. Triglyceride has a higher caloric value than glycogen (9 kcal/g) and being hydrophobic does not have water associated with it. A decrease of 1 g in body fat would require the expenditure of 9 kcal and thus the rate of weight loss after the initial mobilization of glycogen drops dramatically as fat is mobilized. Such fundamental biochemical facts should be carefully explained to the obese patient to avoid disappointment. Complications of starvation diets include hypotension, hypokalaemia, hypomagnesaemia, hyperuricaemia and gout, ketosis, nausea and, if starvation is prolonged, sudden death (see Chapter 2). It is also important to remember that a new body size can only be maintained by chronic control of food intake and often this will involve a change in eating habits to allow the maintenance of a low caloric regime.

Surgery

Surgical intervention is considered only in extreme cases of obesity. Operations such as lipectomy, apronectomy, dental splinting and bowel resection all have associated problems and in any case do not tackle the root cause of the problem. Neurosurgery involving the destruction of the hypothalamic feeding area has now been largely abandoned.

Drugs

Anorectic drugs which appear to act by increasing adrenergic outflow or by inducing a feeling of satiety have been used with partial success. In many cases the drugs have unwanted side effects. Amphetamine which stimulates adrenergic hormone release was commonly prescribed but was withdrawn after side effects of addiction and creation of acute psychotic states became apparent. Fenfluramine has also been used since it induces a state of satiety leading to decreased food intake. However, here again, its side effects of nausea, diarrhoea, excessive dreaming, and precipitation of severe depression on abrupt withdrawal severely limit its use. Although thyroxine increases the basal metabolic rate and would seem therefore an ideal candidate for therapy it is not used unless hypothyroidism exists with the obese state. There is usually an element of thyroxine insensitivity in obesity but use of the hormone promotes loss of lean body mass rather than of adipose tissue. Ideally a molecule which would uncouple mitochondria, in the same way in which brown adipose tissue mitochondria are uncoupled in DIT would be very useful. Dinitrophenol which is a mitochondrial uncoupler was considered for this purpose at one time. This compound was used in the manufacture of explosives and it was noted that some workers in munitions factories became hypermetabolic and suffered a large weight loss. After finding that dinitrophenol was the agent responsible for these effects it was incorporated into commercial slimming preparations. However besides staining the patient yellow there were disturbing side effects and the compound was banned. The search for pharmacological agents which induce thermogenesis in obese subjects continues.

Calcium metabolism

In addition to the calcium requirement for skeletal growth the maintenance of the calcium concentration of intra- and extracellular fluid is critical for a variety of functions. The sole source of calcium is the diet but a rapidly exchangeable pool of calcium in bone whose release is subject to hormonal control is also involved in the maintenance of cellular calcium homeostasis. Under normal conditions humans absorb about 30 per cent of the 900 mg calcium ingested daily and the contribution of dietary calcium to calcium homoeostasis is regulated through hormonal actions on the GI tract and the kidney. The first part of the present chapter will consider the control of intracellular calcium concentrations and the second part the hormonal regulation of extracellular fluid (ECF) calcium homoeostasis.

The control of intracellular calcium

The concentrations of some common cations in extracellular fluid and cell water are given in Table 7.1. The calcium concentration gradient across the

Table 7.1 The distribution of some common cations in extracellular fluid (ECF) and cell water

Cation	ECF (mmol)	Cell water (mmol)
Na$^+$	135–145	12–20
K$^+$	5.3	150
Mg^{2+}	1.1	2.8
Ca^{2+}	3.2	<0.001

plasma membrane is in the same direction as sodium but is much greater; of the order of 10^4, mmol in ECF and probably less than μmol molar in cell water. This difference is maintained by the action of membrane-bound calcium pumps. Calcium is required for a wide variety of processes inside the cell (Table 7.2) and these processes are regulated through changes in the concentration of cytosolic calcium brought about by an influx of calcium from ECF. The sarcoplasmic reticulum of muscle represents an intracellular calcium store which can release calcium to the cytosol in this tissue. Mitochondria also have a large capacity for calcium storage but the

Table 7.2   Some calcium dependent reactions in cells

---

1. Activation of enzyme systems:
   e.g. glycogenolysis, succinate dehydrogenase,
   pyruvate dehydrogenase, α-glycerophosphate dehydrogenase.
2. Inhibition of enzyme systems:
   e.g. pyruvate kinase, phospholipid synthesis.
3. Activation of contractile and motile systems:
   e.g. myofibrils, microtubules, microfilaments.
4. Hormonal regulation:
   e.g. formation of cAMP; hormone release.
5. Membrane linked functions:
   e.g. excitation—secretion coupling in nerve endings.
       excitation—contraction coupling in muscles.
       exocrine secretion.

---

contribution of this organelle to the regulation of cytosolic calcium is not known.

The response of a cell to a particular stimulus, e.g. the binding of a hormone to its specific receptor on the plasma membrane, is often mediated via an influx of calcium into the cytosol and calcium functions as a second messenger of hormone action fulfilling the criteria proposed by Sutherland for such a molecule. However for many of these functions calcium *per se* is inactive and, rather like the effects of cAMP being mediated by the action of cAMP-dependent protein kinases, it is becoming apparent that many calcium dependent regulatory activities in the cell are mediated via a ubiquitous calcium binding protein called calmodulin. This small globular protein (mol. wt. 16 723 = 148 amino acids) has four calcium binding sites and calcium binding increases its α-helical content. It was discovered by chance as an activator of phosphodiesterase during purification of the enzyme. Since the calcium-calmodulin complex can activate the hydrolysis of cAMP and cGMP it can also modulate cyclic nucleotide responsive processes in the cell.

As stated earlier, cell stimulation is often associated with an influx of calcium and, during relaxation, the cation has to be removed from the cytosol to achieve homoeostasis. This involves an ATP-dependent calcium pump which is activated by calmodulin. In most cells this pump is present in the plasma membrane but skeletal muscle also has an intracellular pump which moves calcium into the sarcoplasmic reticulum. The increase in cytosolic calcium in response to a stimulus is detected by calmodulin and as the concentration rises above the K_d* for the calcium-calmodulin complex the complex binds to the pump, activates it and initiates calcium removal from the cytosol. As the calcium concentration falls below the K_d for the complex, it dissociates and no longer activates the pump. In this way calmodulin is able to moderate the intensity and duration of the calcium signal (Fig. 7.1).

A similar picture can be drawn for the activation of other calcium dependent processes, e.g. stimulus-response coupling (Fig. 7.2). Cytosolic calcium rises within milliseconds in response to a stimulus and promotes the

* K_d; dissociation constant for calcium-calmodulin complex.

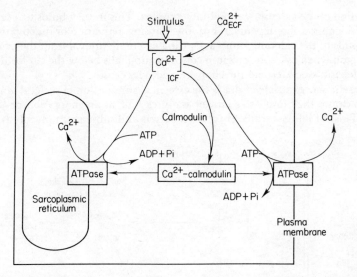

Fig. 7.1 Moderation of intracellular calcium concentration by Ca^{2+}-calmodulin activation of sarcoplasmic reticulum and plasma membrane ATPases.

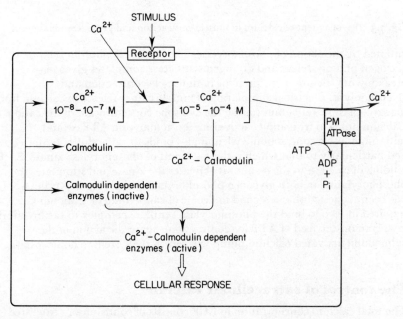

Fig. 7.2 The involvement of calmodulin in stimulus–response coupling. PM–plasma membrane.

formation of the calcium-calmodulin complex. This in turn binds to a series of Ca^{2+}-calmodulin dependent enzymes causing activation or inactivation. It also binds to the calcium pump activating calcium removal from the cytosol and again when cytosolic calcium concentration falls below the K_d for the complex it dissociates and the change in activity ceases.

A particular example of this is the electrical stimulation of skeletal muscle which causes the muscle to contract and uses ATP as an energy source (Fig. 7.3). This ATP is generated by glycogenolysis and subsequent glycolysis

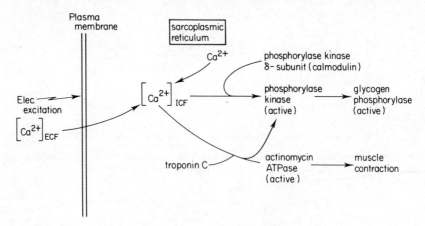

Fig. 7.3 Involvement of calcium in muscle contraction and glycogen metabolism.

initiated by the action of phosphorylase. The reversible phosphorylation of glycogen phosphorylase and glycogen synthetase stimulates glycogen breakdown. Calcium is required for both muscle contraction and glycogenolysis. Electrical stimulation of muscle causes release of calcium from the sarcoplasmic reticulum raising the cytosolic concentration of the cation. Calcium binds to troponin C activating the actomyosin ATPase and initiating muscle contraction. Calcium also binds to calmodulin, both free and particularly to that which is the δ-subunit of phosphorylase kinase. Such binding of calcium to the δ-subunit activates the kinase and stimulates the phosphorylation of both glycogen phosphorylase and glycogen synthetase. It has been suggested that a second molecule of calmodulin or troponin C is required in vivo to bind the phosphorylase-synthase complex to the myofibril giving an on-tap feed of ATP for contraction. Again the action of the calmodulin activated calcium pump will return the system to homoeostasis.

The control of extracellular calcium

The total calcium concentration in ECF consists of contributions from free ionized calcium, that bound to plasma protein and non-ionized calcium salts (e.g. calcium lactate). Since calcium binding to protein (mainly albumin) is dependent on pH this fraction may alter in severe acidosis or alkalosis. The contribution from protein binding will also vary under conditions where

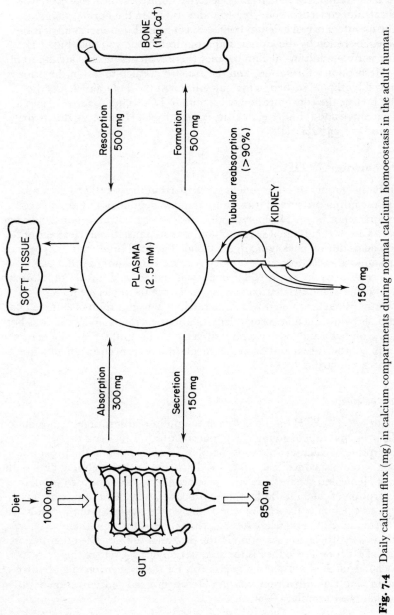

Fig. 7·4 Daily calcium flux (mg) in calcium compartments during normal calcium homoeostasis in the adult human.

plasma protein concentrations are abnormal (e.g. increased in dehydration and myeloma; decreased in chronic renal disease). The physiologically relevant fraction as far as calcium homoeostasis is concerned is the free ionized calcium and a patient may be hyper- or hypo-calcaemic even when total calcium concentration (free + bound) is within the normal range.

The maintenance of calcium homoeostasis in ECF represents a balance between excretion by the kidney and input from bone and gut (Fig. 7.4).

In a normal adult in calcium balance there is no net flux of calcium from bone (resorption = formation) and the amount of calcium lost in the urine is balanced by that absorbed in the gut. Although the daily flux across the tissues is large the concentration of calcium in ECF is maintained within a narrow range and is under endocrine control by PTH and 1,25-dihydroxy$_2$ vitamin D $(1,25(OH)_2D)$.

Parathormone (PTH)

As its name implies this hormone is synthesized in the parathyroid gland where the initial product of translation is a polypeptide of 115 amino acids, preproparathormone. This polypeptide undergoes a cotranslational cleavage of the 25 amino acid signal sequence and a post-translational cleavage of 6 amino acids during packaging in the Golgi. The final product, a polypeptide of 84 amino acids is stored in secretory vesicles. It is of interest that only amino acids 1–34 are required for biological activity and further proteolysis which occurs in the circulation leaves this part of the molecule intact.

Parathormone is secreted when the calcium concentration of extracellular fluids falls below the homeostatic level of about 2.5 mmol and its actions both directly, on bone and kidney, and indirectly, on the gut, serve to increase the calcium concentration and decrease the phosphate concentration of plasma and extracellular fluid.

Actions on kidney

A major effect of PTH on the kidney is to inhibit reabsorption of phosphate in the proximal tubule giving rise to phosphaturia. Effects on the reabsorption of calcium are more complex. Reabsorption in the proximal tubule is diminished while it is increased distally, in the ascending limb of the loop of Henle and the distal tubule. The net effect is an increased tubular reabsorption of calcium. Both of these processes, decreased phosphate and increased calcium reabsorption, contribute to the hypercalcaemic action of the hormone. PTH also decreases bicarbonate reabsorption thereby inhibiting hydrogen ion secretion in the proximal tubule. The other major action of PTH on the kidney is the stimulation, via cAMP, of the mitochondrial 1 α-hydroxylase responsible for the conversion of 25-hydroxy vitamin D to 1,25-dihydroxy vitamin D. A decreased concentration of plasma phosphate has a similar effect.

Actions on bone

Bone represents a huge calcium store and is called upon when exogenous calcium is unavailable. The effects of PTH on bone are complex since they may be different at different concentrations of the hormone. For example, effects on osteoclasts require a concentration of PTH an order of magnitude greater than that required for effects on osteocytes. The initial reponse to the hormone is an influx of calcium into bone cells followed by a stimulation of bone resorption by osteoclasts. Chronically raised levels of PTH may increase the numbers of osteoclasts and high concentrations inhibit bone formation by osteoblasts. The resorptive action on bone coupled with the phosphaturic action on kidney allows a rise in serum calcium to occur without any increase in serum phosphate.

Actions on the GI tract

Parathormone increases intestinal absorption of calcium indirectly through its ability to increase the renal production of $1,25$ $(OH)_2D$. It has no direct action on calcium transport in isolated organ cultures of intestine.

Vitamin D

Although the antirachitic actions of vitamin D have been known for over fifty years the major breakthrough in the understanding of its action was made by De Luca in 1966 who showed that the parent vitamin had to be activated in vivo for biological activity. Vitamin D describes a group of secosteroids the most common being cholecalciferol (D_3) and ergocalciferol (D_2). It is not a true vitamin since it can be synthesized from cholesterol in mammalian skin under the action of sunlight. Only when the daily endogenous production falls below the minimum daily requirement of $5-10\,\mu g$ ($200-400\,iu$) must the balance be met by dietary supplementation. The effects of vitamin D are seen only after activation in the liver and kidney and the final product $1,25$-dihydroxy cholecalciferol satisfies the criteria ascribed to a hormone in that it is synthesized in skin, activated in the liver and kidney and transported to its target tissues, bone and intestine, in the blood (Fig. 7.5). Exogenous vitamin D is absorbed in the duodenum and jejunum from bile salt micelles and appears in the circulation as a constituent of chylomicrons. It is transported to the liver on the chylomicron remnants. The first activation, 25-hydroxylation by a microsomal mixed function oxidase, occurs in the liver and is subject to product inhibition. A second 25-hydroxylase, which is not product inhibited is also present in liver mitochondria and assumes importance in cases of vitamin D intoxication. The product, 25-hydroxy D ($25(OH)D$), circulates bound to a vitamin D binding protein also synthesized by the liver, as the major plasma form of the vitamin with a half-life of about 12 days. The second activation, $1\,\alpha$-hydroxylation by a mitochondrial mixed function oxidase occurs in the kidney and produces the active hormone $1,25$ $(OH)_2D$. The $1\,\alpha$-hydroxylase is activated by PTH and also by decreased intracellular phosphate. As the serum calcium concentration returns to normal and PTH-stimulated $1\,\alpha$-hydroxylase activity decreases, the activity

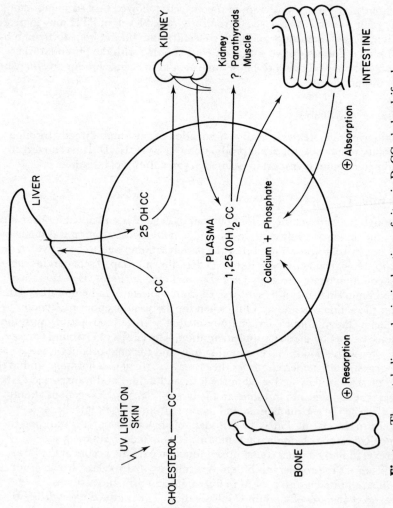

Fig. 7-5 The metabolism and principal actions of vitamin D. CC–cholecalciferol.

of the renal 24-hydroxylase is stimulated and there is increased synthesis of 24,25 $(OH)_2D$. It seems likely that 1,25 $(OH)_2D$ itself stimulates 24-hydroxylation of 25 $(OH)D$ exhibiting a feedback inhibition on the 1 α-hydroxylase. 24,25 $(OH)_2D$ in turn feeds back on the parathyroid gland to inhibit PTH secretion.

Actions of vitamin D

The principal actions of vitamin D are probably mediated via its activated metabolite 1,25 $(OH)_2D$. The major target tissues are bone and intestine although there have been suggestions that the hormone might also affect other tissues (kidney, muscle). The molecule appears to act in a manner similar to other steroid hormones, i.e. it binds to a specific cytoplasmic receptor protein and is transferred to the nucleus where it increases transcription of specific messenger RNA coding for calcium and phosphate transport proteins. In the intestine this leads to increased absorption of calcium at the brush border surface. The ability of the intestine to adapt its absorptive capacity for calcium is dependent on 1,25 $(OH)_2D$. Both dietary and plasma calcium regulate absorption and a need for calcium stimulates the efficiency of intestinal transport. Thus a decrease in plasma calcium stimulates the release of PTH which in turn stimulates the production of 1,25 $(OH)_2D$ in the kidney. A high calcium diet which produces hypercalcaemia has opposite effects on calcium absorption. Intestinal absorption of calcium is against a concentration gradient and movement of the cation from the enterocyte into the circulation at the baso-lateral surface requires sodium ions.

Vitamin D has effects on both bone mineralization and resorption, the latter effects requiring the simultaneous action of PTH. A deficiency of vitamin D leads to defective bone mineralization both during bone growth, which leads to rickets, and also during bone remodelling in the adult which leads to osteomalacia. In each case defective mineralization results from an insufficient supply of calcium and phosphorus to the chondroblasts and osteoblasts. When vitamin D levels return to normal, calcium and phosphate uptake into the cells is enhanced and mineralization proceeds. Resorption of calcium from the labile calcium pool of bone into ECF requires both vitamin D and PTH. Such activity is important in the repair of bone, the maintenance of healthy bone during calcium homoeostasis (bone remodelling) and also in the maintenance of plasma calcium concentration.

Calcitonin

Although many tissues appear to synthesize calcitonin-like peptides the major site of synthesis of immunoreactive calcitonin is the C cells of the thyroid. The circulating hormone consists of 32 amino acids (mol. wt. 3500) but the initial translation product is much larger (mol. wt. 15 000) and includes a signal sequence. Co- and post-translational trimming at both amino and carboxyl terminals occurs to produce the final hormone. In considering the actions of calcitonin it is worth separating physiological and pharmacological actions. Pharmacologically it reduces plasma calcium and inorganic phosphate by actions on bone and kidney and has been of use therapeutically in the treatment of Paget's disease and osteoporosis. Administration of calcitonin inhibits osteoclastic bone resorption and decreases the number of osteoclasts. This leads to a decreased urinary excretion of hydroxyproline and hydroxylysine derived from collagen degradation (of connective tissue). It is possible that the hormone lowers cytosolic calcium in bone cells and thereby decreases efflux of calcium from the pool of labile calcium in the tissue. Its action on kidney to increase the renal clearance of calcium and phosphate may also contribute to its overall effect of lowering the serum concentration of these ions. Although calcitonin inhibits acid secretion in the stomach and stimulates electrolyte secretion into the small intestine it has no effect on intestinal absorption of calcium.

Despite these actions of pharmacological doses of calcitonin the physiological role of the hormone remains to be established. It is tempting to speculate that it is involved in the maintenance of calcium homoeostasis but this has been difficult to demonstrate. Even in the total absence of the hormone as seen in thyroidectomized patients there is no prolonged disturbance of calcium homoeostasis and the patients do not become permanently hypercalcaemic. Lack of the hormone may however give rise to bone loss (osteoporosis) particularly in older women where besides having reduced calcitonin levels there is also a decreased calcitonin response to increases in serum calcium. Very high concentrations of the hormone, as seen for example in patients with medullary thyroid carcinoma, are also well tolerated without giving rise to hypocalcaemia and the inhibition of bone resorption is only temporary. This would suggest that the body adapts rapidly to negate the effects of major changes in calcitonin concentration and that the hormone has no major role in calcium or skeletal homoeostasis. A possible role for the hormone has been suggested recently. The release of calcitonin prior to eating, possibly by gastrin stimulation of the thyroid, would give rise to a transient hypocalcaemia and stimulate the secretion of parathyroid hormone. This in turn would increase the amount of dietary calcium retained by decreasing urinary calcium loss and allow the body to regain calcium homoeostasis during fasting.

The hormone has however been of great value in the treatment of Paget's disease of bone, a condition characterized by increased bone turnover.

Calcium homoeostasis in response to feeding

As previously stated, the concentration of calcium in extracellular fluid is maintained within a narrow range by the actions of PTH, $1,25 \ (OH)_2D$ and possibly calcitonin. When food arrives in the stomach enteric hormones are released and trigger the release of calcitonin from the thyroid. Calcitonin produces a transient hypocalcaemia by inhibiting bone resorption and promoting calcium uptake into a rapidly mobilizable bone pool. Such a transient hypocalcaemia causes the secretion of PTH and allows the body to make maximal use of the incoming dietary calcium load by ensuring complete reabsorption in the renal tubules. The other action of PTH to increase 1,25 $(OH)_2D$ production in the kidney also ensures efficient absorption of calcium from the gut. Thus both kidney and gut act in concert to maintain plasma calcium levels without requiring a net input from bone. Only when there is a prolonged hypocalcaemic stimulus or inefficient calcium absorption from gut is the bone pool called upon. Any excess dietary calcium initially retained by increased reabsorption may then be excreted during the fasting period as the body returns to normo-calcaemia.

Hypercalcaemia

Calcium homoeostasis implies a balance between output in the kidney and input from bone and gut. Hypercalcaemia occurs in response to one or more of the following: (a) increased absorption from the gut; (b) increased net bone resorption; (c) increased renal tubular re-absorption; (d) reduced glomerular filtration rate. Some common causes of hypercalcaemia are given in Table 7.3.

Table 7.3 Some causes of hypercalcaemia and major causes of the maintenance of hypercalcaemia

	Increased tubular reabsorption	Increased bone resorption	Increased intestinal absorption	Renal failure
Primary hyperparathyroidism	+++	+	+	-
Carcinoma with bony metastases (e.g. breast, squamous cell carcinoma of bronchus)		+++		+
Myeloma		+++		+
Vitamin D poisoning	+++	+	++	+
Immobilization (e.g. Paget's disease)		+++		
Tertiary hyperparathyroidism (e.g. due to coeliac disease)	+++	+		++
Sarcoidosis			+++	

+ + + principal mechanism; + + common mechanism; + occasional mechanism.

Severe hypercalcaemia usually involves more than one of the above parameters.

(a) *Increased intestinal absorption.* Conditions such as vitamin D intoxication, sarcoidosis and possibly primary hyperparathyroidism which gives rise to increased concentrations of 1,25 $(OH)_2D$ increase intestinal absorption of calcium by an increase in the calcium and phosphate transport proteins at the brush border surface. Unless dietary calcium intake is very large, however, an increased intestinal absorption alone would produce only a mild hypercalcaemia. Excessive calcium intake may occur in milk-alkali syndrome seen in patients with peptic ulcers who consume vast quantities of milk and also in patients with sarcoidosis. Many of the gut mediated diseases, e.g. sarcoid, cause kidney damage due to increased urinary calcium concentration and stone formation.

(b) *Increased net bone resorption.* Increased bone resorption is a major feature of hypercalcaemia associated with malignant disorders, chronic vitamin D poisoning and immobilization, and is due to the increased actions of both parathyroid hormone and vitamin D metabolites on the tissue.

(c) *Increased renal tubular absorption.* A major effect of PTH is to increase calcium reabsorption in the renal tubules and in primary hyperparathyroidism, over-production of PTH, this produces a mild hypercalcaemia. Ectopic production of PTH or PTH-like substances by tumours especially of the bronchus and kidney may also have a similar effect. The direct actions of vitamin D or its metabolites on tubular reabsorption of calcium are unclear but chronic administration of vitamin D or $1,25\ (OH)_2D$ appear to increase reabsorption independently of PTH.

Hypocalcaemia

Hypocalcaemia is most commonly due to a disturbance in the production or metabolism of, or response to parathyroid hormone and/or vitamin D. Thus the major tissues involved are parathyroid gland, bone, intestine and kidney (Fig. 7.6) and hypocalcaemia arises when intestinal absorption of calcium, renal tubular reabsorption or bone resorption is decreased.

Hypoparathyroidism

This condition may be due to lack of synthesis of PTH after removal or partial removal of the parathyroid gland during neck surgery (e.g. thyroidectomy) or from malignant metastases in the gland. Low levels of PTH cause serum phosphate to rise and calcium to fall as calcium reabsorption in the renal tubules and resorption from bone is decreased. The decreased activity of the PTH stimulated 1-hydroxylation of $25\ (OH)D$ in kidney produces a lowering of serum $1,25\ (OH)_2D$ levels and decreased calcium absorption in the gut. Since the only factor missing is PTH, patients respond to administration of exogenous hormone with a rise in plasma calcium and a phosphaturia. The interaction between parathyroid hormone and vitamin D in hypoparathyroidism is shown in Fig. 7.7.

Pseudoidiopathic hypoparathyroidism

Pseudoidiopathic hypoparathyroidism is due to the synthesis of a defective PTH. The parathyroid synthesizes a product which, although immunologically active is biologically inactive. Thus PTH is detected by

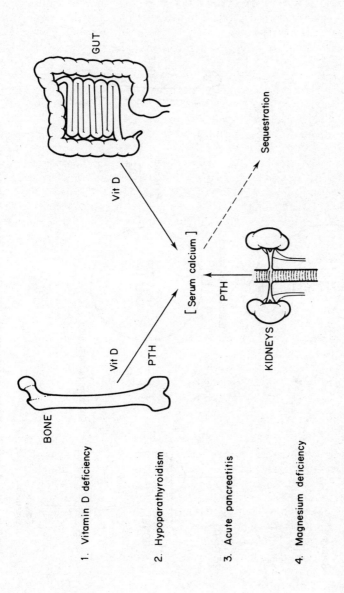

GUT

Vit D

BONE

Vit D

PTH

[Serum calcium]

PTH

Sequestration

KIDNEYS

1. Vitamin D deficiency

2. Hypoparathyroidism

3. Acute pancreatitis

4. Magnesium deficiency

Fig. 7.6 Common causes of hypocalcaemia and the actions of PTH and vitamin D which raise serum calcium.

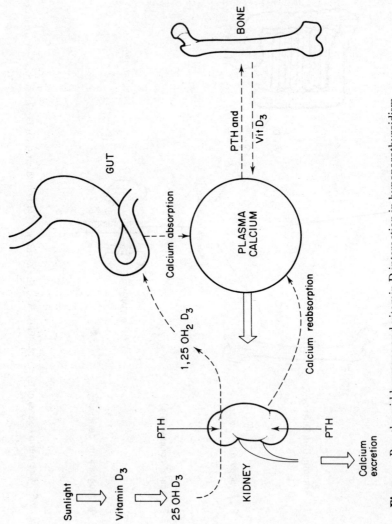

Fig. 7.7 Parathyroid hormone and vitamin D interaction in hypoparathyroidism.

radio immunoassay but patients exhibit hypoparathyroidism since the PTH produced does not initiate responses at its receptors in kidney and bone. Failure to process the initial translated product (125 amino acids) to the active 34 amino acid fragment has not been described but might occur in severe liver disease and produce the same situation. Here, as in hypoparathyroidism, patients respond to exogenous PTH.

Pseudohypoparathyroidism (PHP)

This condition, like hypoparathyroidism (HP) presents with hypocalcaemia and hyperphosphataemia but unlike HP, PTH levels are normal or raised. Patients do not respond to treatment with PTH, i.e. no hypercalcaemia or phosphaturia is seen on administration of exogenous hormone. In such patients the target organs of PTH, bone and kidney, are resistant to the hormone, there being a defect in hormone action rather than secretion. Although some patients show a normal physical appearance others may show short stature, obesity, rounded face, short neck and shortening of the fourth metacarpal or metatarsal bones (Albright's Hereditary Osteodystrophy). The response to PTH in the kidney requires activation of the membrane bound, hormone-sensitive adenyl cyclase and administration of the hormone to a normal individual causes a 50 to 100-fold increase in urinary cAMP within 30 minutes. Such a response requires binding of the hormone to a specific receptor in the kidney plasma membrane and coupling of the hormone occupied receptor to adenyl cyclase on the cytoplasmic face of the membrane. The coupling is performed via the G protein* (guanine nucleotide regulatory protein) which, when hormone binds to the receptor, loses GDP, binds GTP and activates adenyl cyclase. The increased concentration of intracellular cAMP activates protein kinases and stimulates the activity of 25 (OH)D 1 α-hydroxylase to produce 1,25 $(OH)_2D$. A deficiency in any part of this system, e.g. absence of PTH receptors or the G protein, would give rise to a lack of response to PTH. In the latter case (absence of G protein), the patient may present with a metabolic disorder caused by resistance to a variety of hormones whose action is mediated via cAMP. At least seven different disorders of the system presenting as PHP have been described. In some cases the urinary cAMP response may be normal and PHP arises from a failure in the response to the raised cAMP concentration in the kidney. This lack of response to PTH and consequent decreased synthesis of 1,25 $(OH)_2D$ leads to decreased calcium reabsorption in the kidney and decreased absorption in the intestine.

Vitamin D deficiency

A deficiency of 1,25 $(OH)_2D$, the active metabolite of vitamin D, as a result of decreased absorption of dietary vitamin D or impaired production of 1,25 $(OH)_2D$ will also produce hypocalcaemia. Thus those disorders which cause malabsorption of fat, e.g. chronic pancreatitis, diseases of the small bowel,

* More recently this has been termed 'N protein' (nucleotide binding protein).

surgery of the GI tract and diseases which interfere with bile salt production, often produce vitamin D deficiency. In addition, diseases which impair hydroxylations in liver (e.g. chronic liver disease) and kidney (e.g. kidney failure) will result in low levels of 1,25 $(OH)_2D$ and hypocalcaemia. However marked hypocalcaemia is unusual in these cases since low levels of 1,25 $(OH)_2D$ are often compensated by increased production of PTH (secondary hyperparathyroidism).

Magnesium deficiency

Magnesium is required for the release of PTH from the parathyroids in response to a fall in plasma calcium. Hypocalcaemia may be associated with hypomagnesaemia due to impairment of PTH secretion.

Cholesterol metabolism

The prevalence of coronary heart disease as the major single cause of death in the western world (more than 200 000 deaths per year in the UK; double that from cancer) and the general observation that elevated plasma cholesterol is associated with the development of atherosclerosis and coronary heart disease has prompted much research in the scientific world as well as cast cholesterol as an *enfant terrible* in the eyes of popular press. However, cholesterol is an essential component of mammalian cell membranes where it regulates membrane fluidity. It is also a precursor of bile acids in liver, of steroid hormones in sex glands and adrenal cortex and of vitamin D in skin.

Whole body cholesterol homoeostasis

The homeostatic concentration of cholesterol in the plasma, carried by the lipoproteins, is a balance between input from the diet and endogenous synthesis and output via the bile and bile acids (Fig. 8.1). The 'ideal' 70 kg man contains about 140 g of cholesterol of which approximately 8 g (5.7 per cent) is present in the plasma. An 'average' diet contributes about 0.5 g cholesterol each day and endogenous synthesis a further 1 g. As the daily metabolic requirement of cholesterol is around 350 mg the balance has to be excreted via the bile into the faeces. Since practically every cell apart from erythrocytes has the full complement of 26 enzymes required for cholesterol synthesis there is an excessive synthetic capacity in the body and cholesterol homoeostasis necessitates precise regulation of this endogenous synthesis.

Absorption of cholesterol from the gastrointestinal (GI) tract is incomplete and involves cholesterol derived from biliary secretion and desquamated epithelial cells as well as dietary cholesterol. Cholesterol esters in the GI tract are hydrolysed by a pancreatic cholesterol esterase and the free cholesterol partitions into the mixed micelles of bile salts and lipids (monoglycerides, fatty acids and lysophospholipids) from which absorption takes place. A deficiency in bile salt secretion leads to malabsorption of cholesterol. In man, a high cholesterol intake may not necessarily lead to an increase in plasma cholesterol since the body adapts to changes in dietary cholesterol content. On a low cholesterol intake (400–500 mg/day) about 50 per cent is absorbed

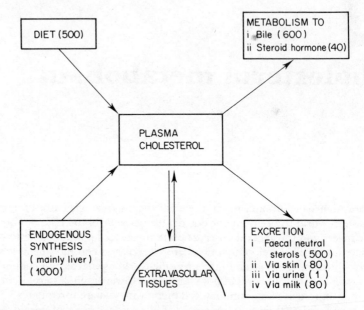

Fig. 8.1   Whole body cholesterol homoeostasis. Figures in parenthesis indicate approximate daily throughput in milligrams.

while on a high intake (1200–1500 mg/day) only about 30 per cent is absorbed. To offset increased input there is an enhancement of neutral sterol excretion in the faeces and decreased endogenous cholesterol synthesis. Once inside the enterocyte the free cholesterol is re-esterified and secreted into lymph as a component of the chylomicron or very low density lipoprotein (VLDL) (p. 79). The entry of dietary cholesterol into the circulation is absolutely dependent on the intestinal synthesis of apoprotein B since without this protein chylomicron and VLDL formation will not occur. In the inherited disorder abetalipoproteinaemia where apo B synthesis is impaired cholesterol and neutral lipid accumulates as droplets in the mucosal cells. Dietary cholesterol eventually reaches the liver as a component of chylomicron remnants or low density lipoprotein (LDL) (p. 79). Although most tissues can synthesize cholesterol only liver and possibly intestine contribute to any significant extent to plasma cholesterol.

Metabolism and excretion of cholesterol

The various routes of cholesterol loss are given in Fig. 8.1. Further metabolism in the liver to bile acids and conjugation with glycine and taurine represents the major loss. Formation of bile acids involves the loss of a three carbon fragment as propionyl CoA (Fig. 8.2). Less than 10 per cent of the bile acid pool is lost daily because bile acids undergo enterohepatic circulation being reabsorbed in the distal ileum. Besides their essential role in micelle formation and lipid absorption in the GI tract bile salts serve as a detergent to keep in solution cholesterol excreted from the liver into the bile.

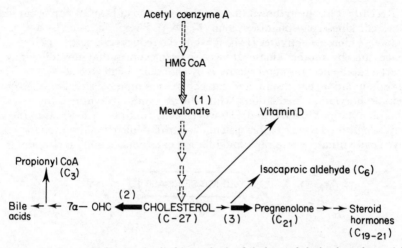

Fig. 8.2 Major control points in the biosynthesis of cholesterol-derived products. (1) 3-hydroxy 3-methylglutaryl coenzyme A reductase (HMGR); (2) cholesterol 7α-hydroxylase; (3) desmolase; 7 α-OHC-7 α-hydroxycholesterol.

Steroid hormone production in the adrenal cortex and sex glands also involves cleavage of the aliphatic side chain of cholesterol (Fig. 8.2). Further detoxication products from steroid metabolism are excreted in the urine. Direct losses of cholesterol occur in the faeces from biliary cholesterol, desquamated cells and non-absorbed dietary sterol. Together with bile acid loss this accounts for 1-1.5 g sterol per 24 hours. Other losses arise as the upper layers of stratum corneum flake off and in the case of the lactating mother as part of the lipid fraction of milk.

Regulation of cholesterol synthesis

Although almost every tissue has the capacity for cholesterol synthesis most research has concerned regulation in liver since this is the major exporter of cholesterol. Cholesterol is synthesized from acetyl CoA via a sequence of 26 steps with the major regulatory reaction at the site of mevalonate production, 3-hydroxy 3-methylglutaryl coenzyme A reductase (HMGR). For instance, cholesterol feeding to rats causes an inhibition of hepatic synthesis of cholesterol from acetate but not from mevalonate and this reflects a parallel inhibition of HMGR but not other enzymes in the pathway. The microsomal enzyme exhibits a diurnal variation in activity in rodents being maximal around the time of major food intake normally at midnight. It has a short half-life of 2-4 hours. Cholesterol feeding of rats causes an inhibition of HMGR activity within six hours probably as a result of modification of existing enzyme while after 24 hours there is a decrease in the amount of enzyme. There is indirect evidence that a diurnal variation of activity also occurs in man (maximum midnight-4 a.m.), and changes in human reductase activity probably do occur in response to dietary cholesterol and hormonal status.

Recently it has been shown that acute regulation of HMGR can occur via a bicyclic kinase/phosphatase system (Fig. 8.3). Phosphorylation by a reductase kinase inactivates HMGR while the reductase kinase is itself inactivated by another kinase. It has also been claimed that hormones may exert a rapid effect on sterol synthesis by changing the degree of phosphorylation, e.g. insulin and catecholamines promote sterol synthesis by dephosphorylation (activation), while glucagon inhibits synthesis by phosphorylation (inactivation). However some controversy exists as to the physiological relevance of this system of control. Unlike the situation for glycogen synthase where rapid modulation of enzyme activity is essential to

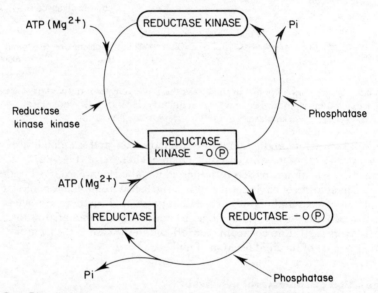

Fig. 8.3   Bicyclic kinase/phosphatase system controlling HMGR.

control glucose levels as intake varies, it is difficult to envisage a physiological situation where the need for such acute control of cholesterol synthesis would be required, particularly in view of the short half-life of the enzyme.

A number of oxysterols e.g. 25-hydroxy- and 7-keto cholesterol are potent inhibitors of HMGR and it is possible that they may serve as physiological regulators in vivo, inhibiting the synthesis and increasing the rate of degradation of the enzyme. In view of the key role of HMGR in the regulation of cholesterol synthesis much research money has been invested on drugs which specifically inhibit the enzyme, particularly for use in the treatment of hypercholesterolaemia. Two such drugs, compactin (ML 236B) isolated from cultures of species of penicillium, and mevinolin, isolated from cultures of aspergillus have received much attention. Both are competitive inhibitors of HMGR and are reported to lower plasma cholesterol (low density lipoprotein cholesterol) in a number of species, including man. In dogs, mevinolin reduced hepatic sterol synthesis by 50 per cent and increased the fractional catabolic rate of LDL by stimulating the synthesis of hepatic LDL receptors thereby lowering plasma and LDL cholesterol concentration. Administration of the drugs leads to an increase in the amount of HMGR in the cell in an attempt to overcome the inhibition caused by the drugs. It is not known what effects prolonged administration of the drug would have in man.

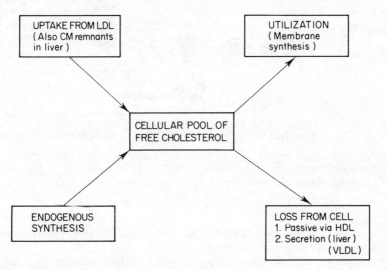

Fig. 8.4 Cellular cholesterol homoeostasis. CH = chylomicron. HDL = high density lipoprotein. VLDL = very low density lipoprotein.

Cellular cholesterol homoeostasis

The cellular pool of cholesterol is also a balance between input into the cell and output (Fig. 8.4). Input includes the uptake of cholesterol from circulating lipoproteins and endogenous synthesis while output includes utilization of cholesterol for membrane synthesis, metabolism to hormones in specialized tissues, and secretion (removal of cholesterol by lipoproteins). When the output is constant, input via lipoproteins and endogenous synthesis bear an inverse relationship. The mechanism by which this occurs was shown by the elegant work of Brown and Goldstein in the USA. Although originally shown for human skin fibroblasts there is good evidence that it obtains for arterial smooth muscle and aortic endothelial cells and may be true for most tissues including liver. The LDL receptor theory is shown in diagrammatic form in Fig. 8.5. The uptake of cholesterol from LDL, the major cholesterol-carrying lipoprotein in human plasma, occurs through two processes.

1. A non specific, low affinity process, bulk phase pinocytosis, where uptake increases linearly in proportion to the extracellular LDL concentration. Cholesterol entering the cell in this way does not regulate

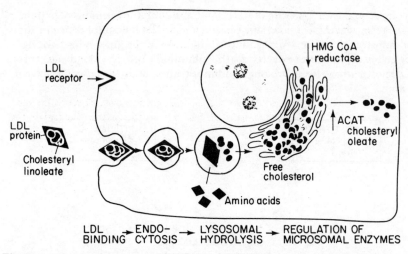

Fig. 8.5   Sequential steps in the LDL pathway in cultured human fibroblasts. (Reproduced from Brown, M. S., Kovanen, P. T. and Goldstein, J. L. (1980). *Ann. N.Y. Acad. Sci.*, **348,** p. 49. New York Academy of Sciences.)

endogenous synthesis of cholesterol. The rate of entry by this process is slow but may become important in atherogenesis.

2. A specific high affinity process, adsorptive endocytosis where uptake is via a LDL receptor on clathrin coated regions on the cell surface. Since the number of receptors on the surface is limited this process is saturable. The rate of cholesterol entry into the cell by this process is much faster than by the low affinity process. Binding of LDL to its receptor via its apo B component causes internalization of the lipoprotein-receptor complex and this is followed by fusion of the internalized vesicle with primary lysosomes. Within the lysosome the apoprotein components of the LDL are hydrolysed to free amino acids while the cholesterol ester is hydrolysed to cholesterol and free fatty acid. The cholesterol is then incorporated in cellular membranes as free sterol. The LDL-receptor probably recycles back to the plasma membrane. Since the cell is able to use this exogenous cholesterol for membrane synthesis, overproduction (accumulation) is avoided by suppression of endogenous cholesterol synthesis at the level of HMGR the rate limiting reaction of cholesterol synthesis. Exactly how this is achieved is unclear since high concentrations of purified cholesterol are required in vitro to inhibit enzyme activity and it is possible that cholesterol derived from LDL via adsorptive endocytosis may undergo oxidation to produce an oxysterol (e.g. 25-hydroxycholesterol) inside the cell which is inhibitory at much lower concentrations. Excess cholesterol entering the cell is stored as cholesterol ester in a reaction catalysed by acylcoenzyme A-cholesterol acyltransferase (ACAT) whose activity is stimulated by LDL-cholesterol. Thus the activities of ACAT and HMGR vary in a reciprocal manner. The number of LDL receptors on the cell surface is strictly regulated to prevent cholesterol

overload in the cell. In the same way that insulin receptor number on the target cell surface decreases as the extracellular insulin concentration increases so the cell adjusts the number of LDL receptors such that the receptor mediated cholesterol uptake from LDL is sufficient for the needs of *de novo* membrane synthesis. As the extracellular LDL cholesterol concentration rises so the number of LDL receptors falls and vice versa.

It should be remembered that in man, where under normal physiological conditions the LDL-cholesterol concentration is in the millimolar range, the number of LDL-receptors on tissues is probably down regulated. Although the low affinity pathway does not normally regulate intracellular sterol metabolism it is probable that entry via these sites contributes more to cholesterol influx than via the high affinity sites.

Transport of cholesterol in the circulation

Transport particles (Table 8.1)

Table 8.1   Major lipoproteins of human plasma

	Chylomicrons	VLDL	LDL	HDL
Density	< 1.006	1.006–1.019	1.019–1.063	1.063–1.21
Diameter (nm)	75–1000	30–80	19–25	4–10
Plasma concentration g/l	1–25	1.3–2.0	2.1–2.5	1–1.5
Electrophoretic mobility	Unchanged	pre-β	β	α
Major components*				
% TG	90	55–65	15	4
CE+C	2–7	10–15	45	17
PL	3–6	15–20	20	24
P	1–2	5–10	20	55
Major apoproteins (% total protein)	ABC (12)(22)(66)	ABC (5)(35)(50)	B (>90)	AC 80–90 5–15 (A-I: A-II) 3:1

* TG—triglyceride; CE + C—cholesterylester + cholesterol; PL—phospholipid
P—protein.
Some properties of the major apoproteins are given in Table 8.2

Chylomicrons (Cm)

Chylomicrons are the lipoproteins of lowest density and are synthesized in the intestine particularly after eating. The triglyceride content and composition reflects the dietary triglycerides which have undergone hydrolysis in the GI tract and resynthesis in the enterocyte. Although the cholesterol content per chylomicron is low (2–7 per cent) the total number of chylomicrons present after a meal, especially a fatty meal, is large and these particles may carry appreciable amounts of cholesterol *in toto*. The apoprotein C–II component is responsible for binding to and activation of the lipoprotein lipase in capillary walls adjacent tò peripheral tissues. As lipolysis proceeds the size of the chylomicron decreases leaving eventually a chylomicron remnant which is sequestered by the liver. The liver does not metabolize whole chylomicrons to any significant extent. Chylomicrons are not normally present in the circulation after an overnight fast.

Table 8.2   Some properties of the major apoproteins

Apolipoprotein	Molecular weight	Major locations	Functions
A–I	28 000	HDL	Cofactor for LCAT
A–II	17 000	HDL	Structural
B	*	CM, VLDL, LDL	Binding to cell receptor
C–II	∼ 10 000	VLDL, LDL, HDL	Cofactor for lipoprotein lipase
D	∼ 20 000	HDL	Cholesterol ester exchange protein
E	∼ 35 000	VLDL, LDL, HDL	Binding to cell receptor; inhibitor of lipoprotein lipase

* There appear to be many different species of ApoB associated with individual lipoproteins.
Values of mol. wt. reported vary between 8000 and 700 000.

Very low density lipoproteins (VLDL)

Triglycerides are also the major component of VLDL which are synthesized mainly in the liver but also the intestine. Progressive loss of triglyceride to peripheral tissues through the action of lipoprotein lipase, again activated by the apo C–II component, causes a gradual increase in density to intermediate density lipoproteins (IDL) and finally low density lipoproteins (LDL). This catabolism of VLDL to LDL involves the loss of apoproteins C and A to high density lipoproteins.

Low density lipoproteins (LDL)

These lipoproteins which are derived from the metabolism of VLDL are the major cholesterol containing lipoproteins in the human circulation. They serve to supply cholesterol to peripheral tissues where they may be destroyed (see p. 78) or return to the liver for destruction.

High density lipoproteins (HDL)

High density lipoproteins represent a spectrum of particles which contain a high proportion of protein with apoprotein A–I and A–II the major protein components. They are secreted by the liver and intestine in a nascent disc shaped form with a high phospholipid to cholesterol ratio. Such discoid particles are seen in large numbers in the plasma of patients with lecithin-cholesterol acyltransferase (LCAT) deficiency. This enzyme (LCAT) binds to the disc and is activated by the apo A–I component. It catalyses the acylation of cholesterol to cholesterol ester with the production of lysolecithin. The hydrophobic cholesterol ester moves to the interior of the particle and eventually generates a spherical particle with a non polar core and a surface film of polar lipids and apoproteins. HDL (typical HDL, HDL—without apo E) contains apoproteins A–I, A–II and C. Since they do not contain apo E they do not bind to the apo B–E receptors of hepatic or extrahepatic tissue. HDL_c (HDL_1, HDL—with apo E) contain apo E in addition to apo A–I, A–II and C and thus bind to the apo B–E receptors in liver and peripheral cells.

Transport of exogenous cholesterol (Fig. 8.6)

After absorption into the enterocyte cholesterol from the diet is incorporated into a chylomicron. This particle is assembled in the Golgi region and consists of a non-polar core surrounded by a monomolecular film of phospholipid and apoproteins A–III and B. In the absence of apoprotein B, secretion into the lacteals does not occur. During passage of the chylomicron to the thoracic duct and into the blood it acquires further apoproteins particularly apoproteins E and C–II from HDL. Apoprotein C–II is a cofactor for the peripheral lipoprotein lipase on the endothelial surface of the blood capillaries. As lipoprotein lipase hydrolyses the triglyceride component to free fatty acid the chylomicron particle becomes smaller and gradually loses apoproteins C–II and A to HDL. Loss of apo C–II decreases the affinity of the particle for lipoprotein lipase and it no longer competes with whole chylomicrons for the enzyme. The change in structure of the particle as triglyceride is lost and also the loss of apo C–II causes a change in location of apo E which is now found on the surface of the chylomicron remnant. The remnant is then recognized by apo E and apo B receptors in the liver parenchymal cells and internalized for destruction by lysosomes. The cholesterol ester is hydrolysed to free sterol which can be excreted via the bile or incorporated in VLDL. Such a transport system is extremely efficient and cholesterol absorbed from the diet does not remain in the plasma for more than a few minutes.

Transport of endogenous cholesterol synthesized in liver (Fig. 8.7)

The assembly and secretion of VLDL in the liver also requires the synthesis of a distinct apoprotein B (different from that in chylomicrons) and the final triglyceride-rich molecule contains cholesterol and apoproteins E and C. Further apoprotein C and E are transferred to VLDL from HDL in the circulation. As in the case of the chylomicron apo C–II is responsible for recognition and activation of lipoprotein lipase and as the triglyceride component is hydrolysed the particle becomes smaller and more dense, losing all apoprotein components except apo B. The resulting LDL is metabolized slowly over a number of days and removed via high affinity apo B/E

82

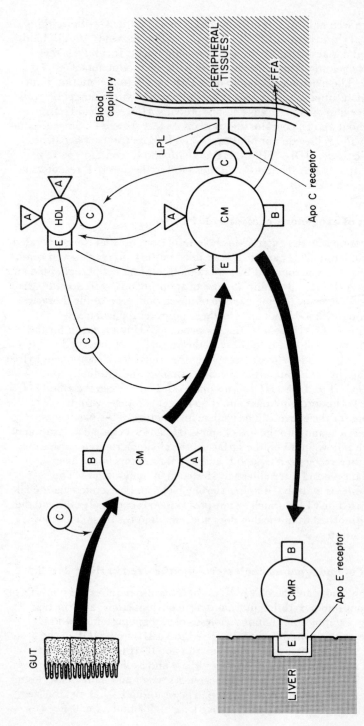

Fig. 8.6 Chylomicron exogenous transport; distribution of dietary fat. (Modified from Havel, R. J. (1982). *Medical Clinics of North America*, **66**, 2, pp. 319–33. W. B. Saunders.) CM = chylomicron. CMR = chylomicron remnant. LPL = lipoprotein lipase. HDL = high density lipoprotein. A, B, C, E = despective apoproteins. FFA = free fatty acid.

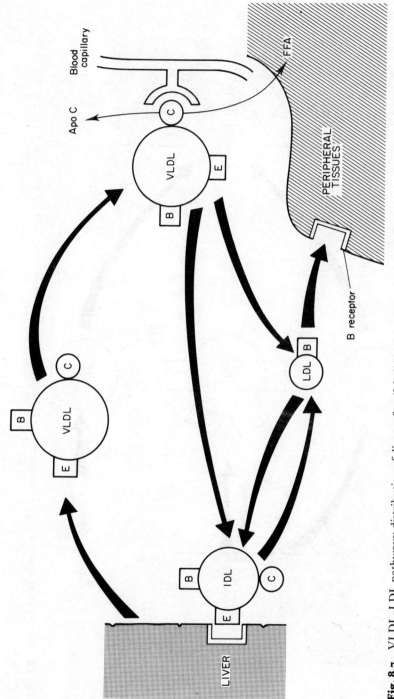

Fig. 8.7 VLDL–LDL pathways; distribution of dietary fat. (Modified from Havel, R. J. (1982). *Medical Clinics of North America*, **66,** 2, pp. 319–33. W. B. Saunders.) IDL = intermediate density lipoprotein.

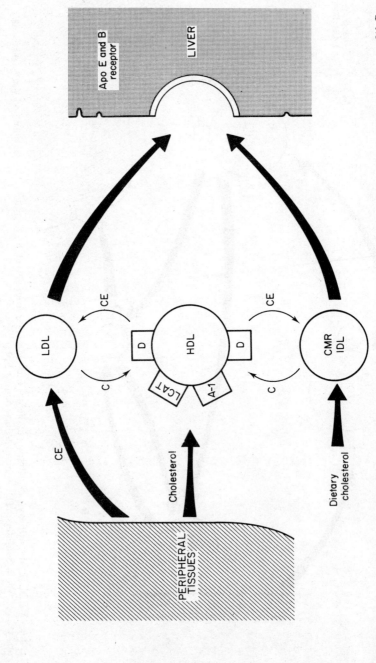

Fig. 8.8 Reverse cholesterol transport. (Modified from Havel, R. J. (1982). *Medical Clinics of North America*, **66**, 2, pp. 319-33. W. B. Saunders.)

receptors in peripheral tissues or liver (see p. 81). A steady state of cholesterol concentration in the cells requires output to equal input so such a delivery of cholesterol to peripheral tissues by LDL must be balanced by a reversed transport system to aid cholesterol efflux. There is good evidence now that HDL plays a crucial role in this process.

Cholesterol efflux from peripheral cells (Fig. 8.8)

From studies using isolated lipoprotein and apoprotein fractions it appears that HDL and in particular apoprotein A–I is the major promotor of cholesterol efflux. Since apoprotein A–II has little effect on efflux it is the small fraction of HDL (5 per cent total) that contains apoprotein A–I not in association with apoprotein A–II that has efflux promoting activity. HDL itself is not secreted in its final form from the sites of synthesis of its protein components (liver and intestine) but as a nascent discoidal particle consisting of bilayers of phospholipid surrounded by protein (apo E and apo A). These apoproteins are also transferred to the particle during catabolism of the triglyceride rich lipoproteins (chylomicrons and VLDL). The cholesterol ester at the core of the particle is derived from the action of LCAT, a component of a small subfraction of HDL secreted by the liver. This subfraction also contains a cholesterol ester transfer component (apo D) which transfers cholesterol ester from HDL to the other lipoproteins, LDL and VLDL. Esterification of the cholesterol in the nascent HDL causes it to change to a spherical shape. The source of cholesterol for the LCAT reaction may be other lipoproteins or, importantly, cell surface membranes. Once the cholesterol ester is formed it is transferred to chylomicron or VLDL remnants and hence may be cleared by the liver via the apo B–E receptors. Sterol ester may also be transferred to HDL to produce a cholesterol rich HDL fraction HDL_c (apo E–HDL) which has acquired apoprotein E and this fraction, normally a small percentage of total HDL, can bind to peripheral or hepatic apo E receptors for clearance from the circulation. In atherogenic hypercholesterolaemia the plasma concentration of normal HDL (without apo E) is decreased while the concentration of HDL_c is markedly raised. Possibly this is a reaction to tissue overload of cholesterol and represents a protective response to clear cholesterol via HDL_c in the liver.

As can be seen from the above it is the apoprotein components of the lipoproteins which determine their metabolism and eventually the fate of the cholesterol that they carry.

Gallstones

Gallstone formation in the gallbladder and common bile duct is a common disease in western society. It is estimated that between 16 000 000 and 20 000 000 Americans have gallstones and in Britain gallstones are found in ten per cent of all necropsies. Although some (25 per cent) of the stones are pigmented precipitates of calcium salts greater than 75 per cent are predominantly crystalline cholesterol monohydrate. The bile is the major excretory route for cholesterol and sterol is maintained in solution by the formation of mixed micelles of lecithin and bile acids. Supersaturation of bile with respect to cholesterol may occur as a consequence of situations which alter the delicate balance of the three lipid classes in bile. For example, increased biliary cholesterol secretion due to increased hepatic cholesterol synthesis or a reduction in the bile acid pool size due to faecal loss or decreased synthesis increase the lithogenicity of bile. In both these instances the liver is at fault and increased HMGR and decreased cholesterol 7 α-hydroxylase activities, the rate limiting steps of cholesterol and bile acid synthesis respectively, have been found in patients with cholesterol gallstones. Supersaturation of bile with respect to cholesterol precedes and predisposes to the formation of cholesterol stones. Increased saturation and a high incidence of gallstone disease is associated with obesity, use of contraceptive steroids and drugs such as clofibrate. As one advertisement states, a major group at risk are the 'fair, female, fat, fertile and forty'.

Precipitation of cholesterol occurs particularly on concentration of bile in the gallbladder. While stones sometimes remain 'silent' and asymptomatic they may obstruct the bile duct causing cholecystitis and produce biliary cholic, fever and jaundice.

At present cholecystectomy is the usual treatment for gallstones both pigmented and radiolucent (cholesterol) and it has been estimated that more than 400 000 cholecystectomies are performed in the USA each year. However, non-invasive treatments aimed at dissolving cholesterol gallstones by desaturating bile have received much attention. Although *de novo* synthesis of cholesterol in the liver accounts for less than one-third of the biliary cholesterol output, inhibition of this synthesis by oral administration of the primary or secondary bile acids, chenodeoxycholic acid or ursodeoxycholic acid (chenotherapy), has achieved some success in dissolution of cholesterol stones. In doses which do not contribute significantly to the total bile acid pool the exogenous bile acids appear to de-activate bile by inhibiting hepatic synthesis and secretion of cholesterol. Gallstone patients treated with chenodeoxycholic acid for six months had lower hepatic HMGR activities than untreated patients. The limited success of bile acids as cholelitholytic agents has prompted investigations into the use of other compounds which inhibit hepatic HMGR. Naturally occurring terpenes such as menthol or their analogues are inhibitors of HMGR in vivo and have been reported to be successful in the dissolution of cholesterol gallstones when used in conjunction with low doses of bile acids. A major problem with such chemotherapy is what happens when the drug is discontinued. Dissolution requires prolonged therapy and in many cases on discontinuation the bile returns to its supersaturated state with the recurrence of gallstones.

Atherosclerosis

Atherosclerosis is the most common lethal disease in western populations. It has no single obvious cause and the major risk factors, hyperlipidaemia, hypertension and cigarette smoking, are not related in any simple way.

Atherosclerosis is a disease of the large and medium sized arteries in which the intima of the arterial wall is thickened by development of fibrous tissue and the accumulation of lipid. Clinical manifestation of the disease mostly results from lesions in the aorta and arteries supplying the heart, brain and lower limbs. The lesions can result in a range of severe diseases caused by gradual occlusion of the artery, sudden occlusion or haemorrhage (Fig. 8.9).

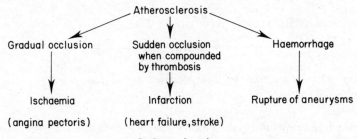

Fig. 8.9 Clinical consequences of atherosclerosis.

The most characteristic feature of developing atherosclerosis is the fibrous plaque, an area of intimal thickening protruding into the lumen of the artery. The thickening consists of an accumulation of fibrous connective tissue containing smooth muscle cells loaded with cholesterol ester and forming an overlay to a larger deposit of extracellular cholesterol ester and cell debris. Complicated lesions, which are the main cause of occlusion of the artery, develop from the fibrous plaques.

Pathogenesis

This is summarized in Fig. 8.10. Initiation (associated with the risk factors mentioned above) is currently thought to result from injury to the endothelial

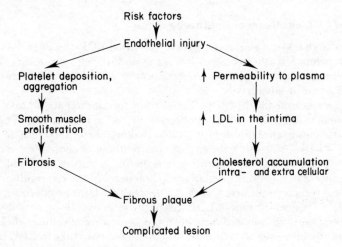

Fig. 8.10 Pathogenesis of atherosclerosis.

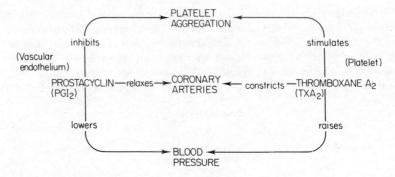

Fig. 8.11   Opposing actions of prostacyclins and thromboxanes on the cardiovascular system.

layer which normally forms the luminal face of the vessel wall. Damage to the endothelium reduces production of prostacyclin (a potent inhibitor of platelet aggregation) and thereby disturbs the normal homoeostatic balance between the opposing actions of prostacyclin and thromboxanes (potent promoters of platelet aggregation synthesized by the platelet by itself (Fig. 8.11). This results in platelet deposition, aggregation, the release of factors causing smooth muscle cell proliferation and eventual fibrosis. The damaged endothelium also shows increased permeability to plasma components which raise the LDL concentration in the intima leading to accumulation of intra- and extracellular deposits of cholesterol ester to complete the formation of the fibrous plaque. Involvement of LDL cholesterol is an essential part of atherogenesis as shown by studies with animal models of the disease. Once it has formed, the raised plaque disturbs normal blood flow making both further damage and thrombus formation more likely. These further events allow growth into a complicated lesion.

Role of LDL cholesterol in atherogenesis

While a large body of evidence correlates elevated LDL-cholesterol levels with occurrence of atherosclerosis it was not until the elegant studies of Goldstein and Brown with human fibroblasts in vitro that a mechanism for the link could be advanced.

   The receptor mediated (high affinity) route for binding and uptake of the LDL particle into cells has already been described in this chapter. The particular importance of this route is that it allows the cell to regulate the uptake of LDL-cholesterol, the endogenous synthesis of cholesterol and the storage as cholesterol ester according to its needs. A feature of critical importance is that overaccumulation of cholesterol in the cell results in decreased receptor numbers and thus a decreased LDL-cholesterol entry rate. At very low concentrations of LDL this pathway accounts for virtually all the cholesterol input to cells and achieves a precise control of cellular cholesterol metabolism. However all cells have also the capacity to take in LDL by a receptor independent, low affinity process resembling non-specific endocytosis. Here the rate of LDL entry is proportional to its concentration up to high values. Both processes result in degradation of the internalized LDL and accumulation of intracellular cholesterol but only the receptor mediated entry is self-regulatory. Accumulation of intracellular cholesterol shuts off entry by the receptor mediated process but does not affect entry by the receptor independent route. Thus at high concentrations of LDL a large part of cholesterol entry to cells is via the uncontrolled low affinity process. Both these routes have now been shown to operate in vivo in animals and man, the receptor mediated route accounting for 33 to 60 per cent of whole body LDL catabolism. Studies in pigs, rabbits and rats show that the organ making the greatest contribution to whole body LDL catabolism is liver at more than 50 per cent of the total rate. In terms of degradation rate per g of tissue liver is also the most active tissue. The contribution of the receptor mediated pathway to LDL breakdown in liver was almost 70 per cent in normal lipaemic rats but in animals made hypercholesterolaemic the contribution of the receptor mediated process was reduced to 39 per cent of the total. Thus in vivo as well as in vitro the receptor mediated route is most prominent in LDL catabolism only at lower LDL concentrations. At elevated LDL concentrations in vivo the resulting down regulation of the high affinity receptor pathway ensures that the receptor independent process contributes an increasingly greater extent to total LDL catabolism.

The importance of the high affinity receptor mediated pathway of LDL uptake and metabolism is amply demonstrated in the case of homozygotes for the genetic disorder familial hypercholesterolaemia. These individuals lack high affinity receptors and as a result catabolism of LDL can only proceed by the receptor independent mechanism, resulting in a decreased fractional clearance rate for LDL and consequently an extremely high plasma concentration of LDL cholesterol. In these individuals the occurrence of atherosclerosis is extremely high, the average age for development of myocardial infarction being around 20 years.

Goldstein and Brown have proposed that the receptor mediated and receptor independent pathways are antagonistic in their influence on atherogenesis. Thus the former pathway functions to protect against the disease while the latter predisposes to it. High plasma concentration of LDL in normal animals and man channels LDL catabolism through the receptor independent pathway and would therefore be associated with atherogenesis.

Most body cells do not obtain LDL directly from plasma but from the interstitial fluid, that is, the ultrafiltrate of plasma through the endothelium. The concentration of LDL in this fluid is around one-tenth that of the plasma. Now studies of human cells in vitro have shown that the maximal percentage contribution of the high affinity receptor mediated pathway to the catabolism of LDL occurs at an LDL-cholesterol concentration of around 0.07 mmol. At higher concentrations the cell's need for cholesterol is exceeded resulting in down regulation of receptors while the receptor independent process is allowing a greater input to occur. Therefore for maximal efficiency of LDL receptor function the plasma LDL cholesterol concentration should be around 0.7 mmol. This happens to be the level of LDL-cholesterol observed in plasma of normal human neonates and animals not subject to atherosclerosis. At this concentration any plasma LDL-cholesterol leaking into the artery wall through areas of damage would be efficiently removed by smooth muscle cells via the high affinity pathway and used for the normal growth requirement of the cell. But even at the mean concentration of LDL cholesterol prevailing in 'normal' western populations (around 3 mmol) the load of LDL-cholesterol presented to smooth muscle cells when plasma leaks into the artery wall is sufficient to exceed the clearance capacity of the receptor mediated process. LDL is therefore taken up by the receptor-independent route leading to an uncontrolled accumulation of cholesterol ester in excess of the cells' needs. The smooth muscle cells now take on the appearance of the foam cells characteristic of atheroma. Further accumulation of cholesterol ester causes toxicity and cell death resulting in the lipid deposits and cell debris that comprise a large part of the fibrous plaque of atherosclerosis. Thus, as a result of dietary and other stresses the increased input of cholesterol in western man exceeds the normal catabolic capacity of the body (mainly the liver) resulting in raised plasma LDL and increased atherogenesis.

Role of HDL cholesterol

As described earlier in this chapter the HDL particle is associated with transport of cellular cholesterol from the peripheral tissues to liver. In this way the HDL particle could be said to be aiding the elimination of body cholesterol since the liver is the major organ for cholesterol excretion. It is therefore significant that an additional risk factor for atherosclerosis is a lowered HDL-cholesterol while longevity is associated with raised HDL cholesterol. However no one has yet shown that raising HDL-cholesterol concentrations in plasma lowers the risk of atherosclerosis, but in vitro studies seem to support strongly a protective role for HDL. Clearly more has yet to be learned about the function of HDL in vivo.

Treatment of atherosclerosis

From what has gone before it is clear that it is raised LDL cholesterol that is the major risk factor associated with the disease. Treatment has concentrated on lowering this by diet (low cholesterol, low saturated fat (to decrease absorption in the gut)), and by drugs such as the bile acid sequestrant cholestyramine. In addition factors associated with raised HDL cholesterol such as regular vigorous physical activity and a lean physique are recommended for those at risk. None of these regimes are particularly efficacious by themselves but it may be significant that recently the mortality due to myocardial infarction in the USA has begun to decline substantially and that country has taken these recommendations seriously for some years.

9

The kidney and hormones

The kidneys are a pair of retroperitoneal organs which lie in the abdominal cavity with their hila at an anatomical level of L_1. They are highly vascularized, deriving their blood supply from the abdominal aorta via the renal arteries and receiving approximately 20–25 per cent (1.1 l.min^{-1}) of the cardiac output. The kidney consists of a medulla and surrounding cortex and under normal circumstances the cortex receives 80 per cent of the renal blood flow. When the renal perfusion pressure lies between 80–180 mmHg the tissue displays autoregulation whereby blood flow in the tissue is kept at a constant rate by vasoactive regulatory mechanisms implemented locally. The kidneys are also highly active metabolically and are involved in many essential functions including:

1. Removal of nitrogenous waste products.
2. Regulation of electrolyte and water balance.
3. Regulation of acid-base balance.
4. Hormone synthesis.

The present chapter describes some of the hormone-sensitive facets of ion and water balance and the role of the kidney as an endocrine organ.

Ion and water balance

The functional unit of the kidney involved in the regulation of ion and water balance is the nephron and each kidney contains 10^6 nephrons equivalent to a tubule length of about 25 miles! Eighty-five per cent of the nephrons lie in the cortex with a further 15 per cent at the cortico-medullary junction. Since approximately 170 litres of glomerular filtrate (GF) are produced each day yet only 1–2 litres of urine are passed an efficient mechanism for modification and reabsorption of the filtrate must exist. The initial filtrate (ultrafiltrate) has a composition similar to that of plasma from which most of the protein has been removed (it still contains some small molecular weight proteins). During passage of the filtrate down the tubule, active reabsorption of solutes such as glucose and protein occurs particularly in the proximal tubule. Reabsorption of such solutes is usually complete and thus they do not appear in normal urine. Their presence in urine usually has pathological significance.

Ions

Although many of the common ions (Na^+, K^+, Ca^{2+}, PO_4^{3-}, NH_4^+, Cl^-). are found in normal urine their concentration is a function of two opposing processes—tubular reabsorption and tubular secretion. The main driving forces for ion exchange are:

1. Active transport (ATP dependent).
2. Passive diffusion down a concentration gradient.
3. Passive diffusion down an electrochemical gradient.

The regulation of sodium concentration

Sodium, at a concentration of 135-142 mmol, is the most abundant extracellular cation and plays an essential role in the maintenance of plasma volume. The fluid content of an average 70 kg man is about 42 litres (60 per cent body weight) of which 60 per cent (28 litres) is intracellular water. The remainder occupies the extracellular compartment comprising blood and interstitial fluid. While water is freely mobile between these compartments, ions are not and water distribution depends on osmotic gradients and membrane permeability. Changes in membrane permeability account for fluid movement which occurs during acute inflammation. An approximate value of the osmotic potential of extracellular fluid may be calculated from the equation:

$$2(Na^+ + K^+) + glucose + urea \simeq 275\text{-}295 \, mOsmol$$

where the concentration of each species is in mOsmol. In this equation sodium, being the major extracellular species is the most important factor. Retention of sodium would lead to an expansion of the extracellular space while sodium depletion would cause a decrease. The consequences of a decrease in circulatory volume would be similar to those of any other hypovolaemic circulatory failure, i.e. tachycardia and hypotension, and if prolonged, tissue anoxia and ischaemia result. This is one cause of pre-renal renal failure. In contrast, sodium, and therefore fluid, retention may cause hypertension and heart failure. Thus regulation of plasma sodium concentration between narrow limits is essential for homeostasis. Sodium excretion via the kidneys is controlled by four major mechanisms. i. distribution of renal blood flow ii. peritubular reabsorption pressure iii. natriuretic factor iv. aldosterone.

Distribution of renal blood flow

Greater than sixty-five per cent of sodium reabsorption occurs in the proximal tubule by the active and passive processes given above Although renal blood flow is directed primarily at the cortex, a redistribution of flow to the medulla, probably brought about by local vasoactive phenomena, increases the number of functioning cortical-medullary nephrons. These nephrons have a very high capacity for sodium reabsorption and thus aid sodium conservation.

Peritubular reabsorption pressure

Alterations in peritubular pressure also increase sodium reabsorption. As the glomerular filtration rate (GFR) changes very little, a decrease in renal blood flow will lead to a relative increase in the protein concentration and thereby increase the osmotic potential of the peritubular fluid. This in turn will affect the movement of water and sodium from the tubule back into the blood.

Natriuretic factor

Natriuretic factor, a hypothetical hormone, has been postulated to act by inhibiting the reabsorption of sodium from the renal collecting ducts and may be secreted in response to an increase in plasma volume. However, its nature and site(s) of synthesis are unknown.

Aldosterone

The major hormonal regulator of sodium reabsorption is aldosterone although other steroid hormones including cortisol and oestrogens may also promote it. Aldosterone is a mineralocorticosteroid produced in the zona glomerulosa of the adrenal cortex. Its principle action is to promote sodium reabsorption and potassium excretion in the distal tubule of the nephron although it also affects sodium transport into other body fluids such as saliva. Only about 10 per cent of the initial sodium load reaches the distal tubule and aldosterone regulates the distribution of 20 per cent of this (i.e. 2 per cent of the total sodium load). Although this appears to be a very small proportion of the total load, if one considers a GFR of 180 litres/day and a sodium concentration of 140 mM then in the absence of aldosterone action there is a potential loss of 504 mmol Na^+ ($180 \times 140 \times 0.02$) per day, equivalent to 30g of table salt. Thus aldosterone acts as a fine regulator of sodium excretion. Patients whose adrenals have been removed and are unable to synthesize the hormone may become severely sodium depleted and hypotensive if untreated.

As with other steroid hormones aldosterone binds to cytosolic receptors in target cells and the receptor-hormone complexes enter the nucleus where they bind to DNA and promote the synthesis of specific mRNA. This mRNA is then translated into specific protein molecules which mediate the cellular response to the hormone. Aldosterone stimulates the synthesis of a specific sodium/potassium transport protein in the kidney but since this process takes about 45 minutes it is likely that the hormone has chronic rather than acute actions on sodium excretion.

Factors regulating aldosterone secretion

(a) Adrenocorticotrophic hormone (ACTH). ACTH in high concentration stimulates the release of aldosterone but the physiological significance of this is unknown.

(b) Plasma sodium and potassium. Aldosterone secretion is stimulated directly by a fall in plasma sodium or a rise in plasma potassium and leads to a return to homoeostasis by increasing tubular reabsorption of sodium and excretion of potassium. This is a good example of simple feedback regulation.

(c) Renin-angiotensin system. This is probably the major regulator of aldosterone release. Renin, a glycoprotein (mol. wt. 42,000) is synthesized and stored as an inactive proenzyme in cells of the macula densa of the distal convoluted tubule. Stimulation of renin release (see below) results in the liberation of an active proteolytic enzyme which hydrolyses angiotensinogen, an α_2-globulin synthesized in the liver, to angiotensin I. This primary product has little intrinsic biological activity until it is further hydrolysed to angiotension II, an octapeptide, by the action of converting enzyme. Converting enzyme is present in high concentration in lung parenchymal tissue but it is also widely distributed on the vascular endothelium of other tissues and local production of angiotensin II may be physiologically important. However, the principle site of converting enzyme activity seems to be in the lung. Further hydrolysis of the N-terminal aspartic acid of angiotensin II by an aminopeptidase produces a heptapeptide, angiotensin III. Angiotensin II has a short plasma half life of 1–2 minutes, being rapidly destroyed by angiotensinase. Its major actions are twofold:

1. It is a powerful vasoconstrictor and thereby plays an important role in the maintenance of blood pressure.
2. It acts on the adrenal cortex to promote aldosterone release.

The plasma half life of angiotensin III is also of the order of 1–2 minutes. Although it is not such a powerful pressor agent as angiotensin II it has a pronounced effect on aldosterone release. The presence of an amino peptidase in the adrenal cortex which acts as a local converter of angiotensin II→III suggests that angiotensin III may be an important stimulator of aldosterone release.

The regulation of sodium excretion is, in essence, the regulation of plasma volume as illustrated by factors which stimulate renin release, i.e. i. reduced renal perfusion pressure, ii. adrenergic outflow, iii. reduced tubular sodium. A fall in blood pressure would lead to a reduction in renal blood flow and, systemically, to an adrenergic drive to stimulate peripheral vasoconstriction. Both of these events would promote renin release and thus (a) increase sodium reabsorption causing an expansion in plasma volume and (b) stimulate angiotensin synthesis and produce a vigorous vasoconstriction in an attempt to restore blood pressure (Fig. 9.1). A consequence of sodium retention via aldosterone action on the kidney is potassium excretion.

Clinical aspects

Adrenal hyperfunction, as seen in Cushing's disease, may lead to excessive sodium retention and consequent hypertension. Similarly the hypertension associated with oestrogen contraception is probably due to sodium retention. Conversely, adrenal hypofunction (e.g. Addison's disease) is associated with a decrease in plasma sodium and an increase in plasma potassium. This may be manifest as severe hypotension and liability to cardiac arrhythmias.

Cardiac failure may result from inappropriate physiological regulation. A

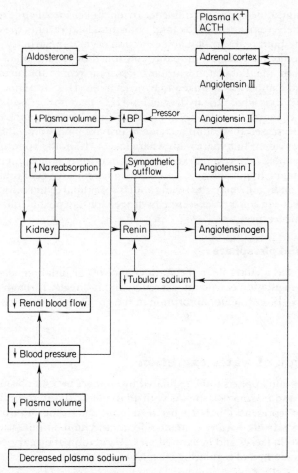

Fig. 9.1 The regulation of plasma sodium concentration and its interrelation to plasma fluid volume.

fall in cardiac performance produces a fall in systemic perfusion pressure and a consequent fall in renal perfusion pressure stimulates sodium and water retention so expanding the plasma volume. This increase in plasma volume imposes an extra work load on the heart (by dilating the ventricles such that they do not contract efficiently) and aggravates the cardiac failure reducing still further the cardiac output. This vicious circle may prove lethal if not broken. A reduction of plasma volume by the administration of diuretics, which override inappropriate self-regulatory mechanisms, can produce dramatic results.

Potassium

Potassium excretion is controlled only partially by aldosterone action on the kidney. As with sodium, most of the potassium reabsorption takes place in the proximal tubule under the influence of ion and electrochemical gradients. Approximately 10 per cent of the total potassium load reaches the distal tubule where both reabsorption and excretion occur. The urinary concentration of potassium is probably controlled by regulation of excretion in the distal tubule. Potassium transport across the renal tubular membrane is closely and competitively linked to hydrogen ion (H^+) excretion. In metabolic acidosis where the hydrogen ion [H^+] load is increased potassium excretion is reduced. Conversely, in metabolic alkalosis where the hydrogen ion load is decreased there is an increase in urinary potassium. This is particularly evident in hyperemesis where loss of H^+ in the vomitus creates a metabolic alkalosis. Here a marked increase in urinary potassium creates a reactive systemic hypokalaemia. Similarly, in hereditary renal tubular acidosis, a condition where the renal tubules seem unable to reabsorb bicarbonate, or in some cases secrete hydrogen ions, hypokalaemia is a characteristic feature.

Calcium and phosphate

The kidney has a vital role in the maintenance of calcium homoeostasis both directly by regulation of calcium excretion and indirectly through the action of $1,25\,(OH)_2D$ on calcium absorption in the gut. This is discussed more fully in Chapter 7.

Regulation of water excretion

Water excretion appears to be regulated by changes in both plasma osmolarity and plasma volume. As with all dynamic states in equilibrium, the steady state represents a balance between input and output, in this case fluid intake (water drunk + water content of food) and fluid output (water lost as urine, sweat, in faeces and in expired air). Regulation of urinary volume is the obvious method of regulating output (Fig. 9.2).

Urinary output

Most of the water in the ultrafiltrate is reabsorbed in the proximal tubule as a result of imposed osmotic gradients and less than 10 per cent of the initial glomerular filtrate reaches the distal tubule. Since the absorption profile of all the components of the original filtrate is similar, the osmolarity of the fluid in the distal tubule is approximately 150 mOsmolar, i.e. hypotonic with respect to plasma. It is the reabsorption of water present in the distal tubule which is subject to regulation by antidiuretic hormone (ADH). Antidiuretic hormone (vasopressin) is an octapeptide synthesized in the neurones of the supraoptic hypothalamic nuclei. It is bound to a protein (neurophysin II) and transported by axonal flow to the terminal bulbs of the neurones in the posterior pituitary. Release of the hormone from the posterior pituitary is stimulated by an increase in the osmolarity of blood perfusing the hypothalamus (direct stimulation) and inhibited by an increase in plasma volume detected by baroreceptors in the left atrium.

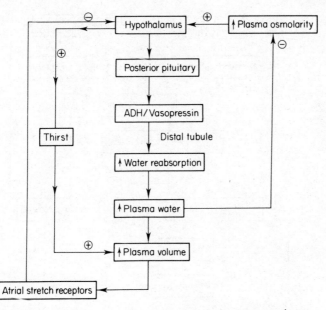

Fig. 9.2 Regulation of plasma osmolarity via control of water excretion.

ADH acts primarily on the distal tubule increasing tubular permeability. It binds to specific receptors on the tubular membrane and increases intracellular cAMP concentration by activating adenyl cylase. Tubular permeability is increased as a result of increased dilation of membrane pores. There is evidence to suggest that the number of pores may also be increased. Water then moves according to the existing osmotic gradient and the osmolarity of urine may be raised to 1000 mOsmolar under the influence of the hormone. In addition to these actions ADH also has a minor vasoactive role, causing vasoconstriction of arteriolar and capillary beds, one consequence of which is to decrease renal blood flow. As mentioned earlier (see p. 93) a decreased renal blood flow with a constant GFR may lead to increased water absorption in the proximal tubule by increasing the osmotic potential of the peritubular fluid.

Osmolarity can also be influenced by water intake. Decreased plasma volume, usually associated with an increased plasma osmolarity, also serves to raise the plasma concentration of angiotensin II. This molecule appears to have a powerful stimulatory effect on the thirst centre (Fig. 9.3).

Clinical aspects

Diabetes insipidus, a disease characterized by the production of large volumes of dilute urine, has two main aetiologies:

1. Decreased production of ADH by the posterior pituitary e.g. due to carcinoma or after trauma.
2. An inborn error in which the renal tubules are insensitive to ADH.

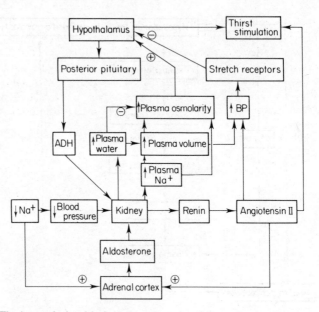

Fig. 9.3   The interrelationship between plasma sodium concentration and plasma water.

Prolonged diuresis leads to dehydration, hypotension and a state of hypernatraemia. ADH action can also be inhibited by a number of drugs including alcohol which has a marked inhibitory effect on posterior pituitary function and may explain the diuresis which accompanies alcohol consumption.

Over production of ADH due to a pituitary tumour or more usually to oat cell carcinoma of the bronchus results in the formation of an extremely concentrated urine. Excessive water retention eventually leads to water intoxication and massive electrolyte imbalance.

Renal hormone synthesis

Renal erythropoietic factor (erythrogenin; REF)

Erythropoiesis is stimulated by erythropoietin, a globular glycoprotein (mol. wt. 40 000) synthesized in the liver. It is present in the circulation in an inactive form. Activation of the pro-hormone is mediated by a proteolytic modification catalysed by a factor synthesized in the kidney, renal erythropoietic factor or erythrogenin. The activated erythropoietin has a plasma half life of about 5 hours. Such an activation is analogous to the renin-angiotensin system but none of the proteases of this system appear to be involved in erythrogenesis. The cellular site of REF synthesis has not yet been established although it has been suggested that cells of the juxta glomerula complex and the glomeruli might be involved. Production of REF, like that of erythropoietin is stimulated by hypoxia, alkalosis and β-adrenergic drive. Cobalt ions and androgens also stimulate REF production. The interrelationship of hepatic and renal factors is shown in Fig. 9.4.

Renal damage may lead to decreased REF production with a consequent anaemia and may account for anaemias seen in chronic renal failure. On the other hand, renal tumours may give rise to raised REF production producing a reactive polycythaemia.

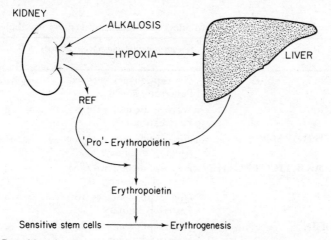

Fig. 9.4 Renal involvement in the control of erythrogenesis.

Vitamin D activation
The hydroxylation of 25-OH vitamin D to its active metabolite $1,25\ (OH)_2D$ is considered in Chapter 7.

Prostaglandin synthesis
Recent evidence suggests that the kidney is a very active producer of prostaglandins especially PGI_2 and PGE_2. These may be involved in the control of renin release and systemic blood pressure. A detailed discussion of this is beyond the scope of this chapter.

Thus the kidney is not merely an organ developed for waste disposal, it is an extremely active tissue which is the target of a host of interrelated endocrinological controls serving as an important source of hormones which control a range of functions including blood pressure, erythrogenesis and calcium metabolism.

Appendix

The appendix contains four tables which summarize the sites of synthesis and major metabolic effects of hormones referred to in earlier chapters.

Table A1. Properties of some hormones controlling intermediary metabolism

Hormone	Chemical nature and site of synthesis	
INSULIN	Polypeptide mol. wt 5000 Pancreatic β-cells	= 51 amino acids
GLUCAGON	Polypeptide mol. wt 3485 Pancreatic α-cells	= 29 amino acids
GROWTH HORMONE	Polypeptide mol. wt 27 000 Anterior Pituitary	=191 amino acids
ADRENOCORTICOTROPHIN	Polypeptide mol. wt 4500 Anterior Pituitary	= 39 amino acids
VASOPRESSIN	Oligopeptide mol. wt 1000 Posterior Pituitary	= 9 amino acids
OXYTOCIN	Oligopeptide mol. wt 1000 Posterior Pituitary	= 9 amino acids
PARATHORMONE	Polypeptide mol. wt 9500 Parathyroid	= 84 amino acids
THYROTROPHIN	Polypeptide mol. wt 28 300 Anterior Pituitary	= amino acids
CALCITONIN	Polypeptide mol. wt Thyroid 'C' cells	= 32 amino acids
THYROID HORMONE	Amino acid derivative mol. wt Thyroid	$T_3 = 651$ (mol. wt) $T_4 = 767$ (mol. wt)
PROLACTIN	Polypeptide mol. wt 22 000 Anterior Pituitary	=199 amino acids
GLUCOCORTICOID	Steroid Adrenal cortex (zona glomerulosa)	
MINERALOCORTICOID	Steroid Adrenal cortex (zona fasciculata)	
CATECHOLAMINES	Amino acid derivatives chromaffin tissue, adrenal medulla	

Homoeostatic blood concentration	Major target tissues
0.5–0.8 ng/ml (10–20 uU/ml)	Liver, adipose, muscle
75–150 pg/ml	Liver, adipose
	Liver, adipose, muscle
6 a.m. 10–50 pg/ml 6 p.m. 10 pg/ml	Adrenal cortex
0.4–0.8 pg/ml (1–2 uU/ml)	Kidney
	Smooth muscle of uterus and mammary gland
0.73 ng/ml	Kidney, bone
5 μU/ml	Thyroid
100 pg/ml (fasting)	Bone, kidney
T4 50–130 ng/ml	Muscle, liver, kidney
T3 0.8–1.8 ng/ml	
	Mammary gland, ovaries, testes, kidney, fetal lung
Cortisol 8 a.m. 50–150 ng/ml	Muscle, liver, adipose
Aldosterone 0.03–0.1 ng/ml	Kidney
Adrenaline 0.02–0.04 ng/ml Noradrenaline 0.2–0.4 ng/ml	Cardiovascular system, muscle, adipose, pancreas (liver), thyroid, parathyroid, kidney

Table A2 Some metabolic effects of insulin and glucagon

Insulin	Glucagon	Process	Tissue
↑		Glucose uptake	Muscle, adipose
↑(both)	↓(liver)	Glycogen synthesis	Muscle, liver
↓(both)	↑(liver)	Glycogenolysis	Muscle, liver
↓	↑	Gluconeogenesis	Liver, kidney
↥(muscle)	↑(liver)	Amino acid uptake	Muscle
↑		Protein synthesis	Muscle
↑	↓	Lipogenesis	Adipose, liver
↓	↑	Lipolysis	Adipose
↓	↑	Ketogenesis	Liver

Table A3 Major metabolic actions of cortisol on carbohydrate, protein and fat

Carbohydrate	↑Gluconeogenesis
	↑Peripheral antagonism to insulin
Protein	↑Degradation↓synthesis in muscle
	↑Concentration of circulating amino acids
	↑Synthesis of gluconeogenic enzymes in liver
	↑Ureogenesis
Fat	Hyperlipaemia; hypercholesterolaemia;
	Centripetal distribution of fat

Table A4 Some metabolic effects of catecholamines

Tissue	Effect	Result
WHOLE BODY	↑Thermogenesis	↑metabolic rate
LIVER	↑Glycogenolysis	} ↑glucose output
	↑Gluconeogenesis	
	↑Ketogenesis	↑ketone body output
	↑K^+ uptake	↑maintains K^+ homeostasis
ADIPOSE TISSUE		
(White)	↑Lipolysis	↑blood FFA
(Brown)	↑Lipolysis	↑local thermogenesis
MUSCLE	↑Glycogenolysis	↑lactate output
	↓Glucose uptake	↑blood glucose
	↑Ca^{2+} uptake	↑contractile strength
	↑K^+ uptake	
KIDNEY	↑Gluconeogenesis	↑glucose and ammonia output
	↑Free water clearance	↑urine output
	↑Na^+ reabsorption	↑ECF
	↑Ca Excretion	Hypercalciuria

Index